Functional
Assessment of
Low Vision

Functional Assessment of Low Vision

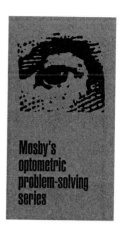

Mosby's
optometric
problem-solving
series

Edited by

Bruce P. Rosenthal
OD, FAAO

The Lighthouse, Inc.
111 East 59th Street
New York, New York

Roy Gordon Cole
OD, FAAO

State University of New York
State College of Optometry
100 East 24th Street
New York, New York

Series Editor

Richard London, MA
OD, FAAO

Diplomate, Binocular Vision and Perception
Pediatric and Rehabilitative Optometry
Oakland, California

with 78 illustrations

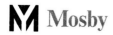 Mosby

St. Louis Baltimore Boston Carlsbad Chicago Naples New York Philadelphia Portland
London Madrid Mexico City Singapore Sydney Tokyo Toronto Wiesbaden

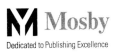

Mosby

Dedicated to Publishing Excellence

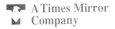

A Times Mirror
Company

Executive Editor: Martha Sasser
Developmental Editor: Kellie F. White
Project Manager: John Rogers
Design Coordinator: Renée Duenow
Series Design: Jeanne Wolfgeher
Manufacturing Manager: Theresa Fuchs

Printed in the United States of America
Composition by Shepherd, Inc.
Printing/binding by Plus Communications

ISBN 0-8151-7347-4

Mosby–Year Book, Inc.
11830 Westline Industrial Drive
St. Louis, MO 63146

95 96 97 98 99 / 9 8 7 6 5 4 3 2 1

Contributors

Aries Arditi, Ph.D., FAAO
Director, Vision Research
The Lighthouse, Inc.
New York, New York

Sherry J. Bass, OD, FAAO
Professor
State University of New York
State College of Optometry
New York, New York

Roy Gordon Cole, OD, FAAO
Diplomate in Low Vision
Chief Low Vision Service
State University of New York
State College of Optometry
New York, New York

Eleanor E. Faye, MD, FACS, FAAO
The Lighthouse, Inc.
New York, New York

Michael L. Fischer, OD, FAAO
Director of the Low Vision Service
The Lighthouse, Inc.
New York, New York

Arthur Ginsberg, Ph.D.
Director of Research and Development
Vision Sciences Research Corporation
San Ramon, California

E. Eugenie Hartmann, Ph.D.
The Lighthouse, Inc.
New York, New York

Kenneth Knoblauch, Ph.D.
Cerveau et Vision
Bron, France

Bruce P. Rosenthal, OD, FAAO
Diplomate in Low Vision
Chief Low Vision Programs
The Lighthouse, Inc.
New York, New York

Jerome Sherman, OD, FAAO
Distinguished Professor
State University of New York
State College of Optometry
New York, New York

To our wives Susan and Carol and children Jason, Kerrin, and Andrew and Jason, Matthew, and Daniel

To Dr. Barbara Silverstone for her continuing leadership and support in bringing low vision into the 21st century. To the Lighthouse, Inc. staff in New York who devote 100% of their energy towards direct service, research, and continuing education of individuals with a visual impairment. It is a great pleasure to work with all of these talented people.

To the State University of New York College of Optometry Low Vision Service Staff who provide the highest level of patient care, innovative lens design, and excellence in instruction to the Optometry students at the college.

To Richard Feinbloom who has always been there to carry out a low vision idea.

To Drs. Robert Rosenberg and Frank Brazelton who ignited our interest in low vision.

Preface

The professions of Optometry and Ophthalmology have seen extraordinary advances and changes during the past two decades. The use of diagnostic and therapeutic pharmacological agents have forever altered the Optometric management of patients while innovative surgical techniques, ophthalmic materials, and high tech instrumentation have profoundly affected Ophthalmological care.

In the United States, in a span of less than two decades we have witnessed such changes as:

- the demise of the aspheric aphakic correction and large surgical keyhole pupils following cataract surgery;
- the improved medical management and treatment of the person with hypertension or diabetes;
- the versatility and myriad uses of the ophthalmic laser.

All of these changes have resulted in the early detection and management of ocular diseases such as: macular degeneration, glaucoma, cataract, and diabetic retinopathy. This, in turn, has resulted in markedly improved functional vision. New techniques that will be commonplace in Optometric/Ophthalmologic practices in the 21st century will uncover pathology at even earlier stages. For example, it is likely that, within the next few years, diabetics and individuals with high cholesterol will be readily detected by Optometrists and Ophthalmologists using noninvasive techniques.

Advances in medical care and surgery will translate into growing numbers of individuals who will require the services of clinicians well versed in low vision evaluation and remediation. The "baby boom generation" will also be going through a transformation from the middle-aged to older-aged. This is the first generation to pay attention to the dangers of smoking, and give more notice to diet and exercise. Theoretically this concern for a healthier body should translate into larger numbers of individuals surviving into their 80's, and 90's, and beyond. Concurrent with this growth in the older population will be a significant increase in the number of individuals who will require the services of low vision specialists.

With these changes in mind, the authors have developed two separate texts. This text will deal with the Functional Assessment of Low Vision while the second book will be concerned with Remediation and Management of Low Vision Problems.

Functional assessment tools such as the measurement of visual acuity, visual field, contrast sensitivity, and color perception make up the essential elements of the current low vision evaluation. Rosenthal, Cole, Hartman, Faye, Ginsburg, Bass, Fischer, Arditi and Knoblauch will cover the essentials of low vision assessment for the adult and child. Completing the assessment will be specialized techniques by Sherman.

Low vision care should continue to expand at the phenomenal rate that has existed for the past 20 years. The authors hope that the work of Feinbloom, Faye, Hellinger, Rosenberg, Mehr, Freid, Hoeft, Bailey, Jose, and Freeman will continue to inspire clinicians into the 21st century.

We hope that this book adds to the impressive works that have already been published by Faye, Mehr and Freid, Nowakowski, Cole and Rosenthal, Jose and Freeman, Newman, Sloan, Fonda, and Bier.

Acknowledgments

We would like to thank Kellie White for the endless time devoted to our manuscript. Thanks also to Martha Sasser, Amy Dubin and the others at Mosby for all the work that they have put in on the manuscript. To Dr. Rick London who has been kind enough to consider our books for his series.

A special thanks to Karen Seidman for all her help in the preparation and proofreading of the chapters.

To the contributing authors without whose help this book could never have been written.

Bruce P. Rosenthal
Roy Gordon Cole

Contents

1

The Function-Based Low Vision Evaluation

Bruce P. Rosenthal

Key Terms

Visual function	Contrast sensitivity	logMAR
Visual acuity	Amsler grid	Intake history

The emphasis in managing a low vision patient has changed dramatically during the past 30 years. There has been a shift away from optics and low vision devices toward visual function. This movement began with the writings of Mehr and Freid,[1] Faye,[2] and Newman[3] in the late 1960s and early 70s and continued into the 80s and 90s when Faye,[4] Rosenthal and Cole,[5] Cole and Rosenthal,[6] Freeman and Jose,[7] and Nowakowski[8] began to underscore the importance of visual function testing in the assessment of patients.

The approach to low vision patient management was also undergoing a transformation during this period. Today the management of low vision patients may be thought of as a continuum, beginning with surgical and medical intervention and proceeding through to the prescription of low vision device(s) and necessary rehabilitative services.

The current concept of low vision patient management is that treatment—whether medical, optical, or rehabilitative—can take place on parallel tracks. For example, medical intervention (e.g., the treatment

1

CLINICAL PEARL

Today the management of the low vision patient can be thought of as a continuum, beginning with surgical and medical intervention and proceeding through to the prescription of low vision device(s) and necessary rehabilitative services.

of chronic open-angle glaucoma) can take place simultaneously with the prescription of optical devices to maximize residual vision along with other intervention strategies. These might include training by an orientation and mobility specialist as well as job-site intervention. The ultimate outcome is to enhance the individual's ability to function as close to the norm as possible, using a variety of strategies.

CLINICAL PEARL

The ultimate outcome is to enhance the individual's ability to function as close to the norm as possible, using a variety of strategies.

Functional Tests

Changes in the low vision examination began as early as 1970, when Faye[2] recommended inclusion of the Amsler grid in the low vision battery. However, instead of using the Amsler grid primarily as a diagnostic indicator of central vision loss, she suggested it could become a predictor of success with low vision devices. Emphasis was placed on the integrity of the grid and the position, density, and size of the scotomas. She also suggested that clinicians look at how the ocular pathology affected the prescription, acceptance, and ultimate success of low vision devices.

Sloan[8] introduced the first set of standardized visual acuity charts with M notation in 1959, and Bailey and Lovie[9,10] made further modifications with the logMAR chart in 1976. Bailey & Lovie recommended using a chart that had letters of equal legibility, the same number of letters in each row, and uniform letter and between-row spacing. They also advocated that there should be a "logarithmic progression of letter size." This was followed by their development of a near vision chart, in 1980, that used unrelated words arranged in a logarithmic progression of size. The charts were intended to be used for the systematic assessment of reading acuity and visual efficiency. Ferris et al.[11] proceeded to use the Bailey-Lovie chart for clinical research, which resulted in acceptance of the "Ferris-Bailey" chart (Fig. 1-1) for all such endeavors by the low vision community. In other articles Bailey[12,13] called for an additional change in visual acuity measurement, the elimination of Jaeger and reduced Snellen notation and replacing it with the logMAR (log of the minimum angle of resolution) system.

In the 1980s the ETDRS single-letter chart (Fig. 1-2) was further modified for near and introduced into the Lighthouse battery[14] along with standardized continuous adult (Fig. 1-3) and child text reading cards. These cards are primarily used for predicting the dioptric power necessary to achieve a patient's objective.

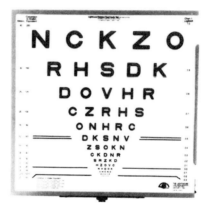

FIGURE 1-1 The Ferris-Bailey chart.

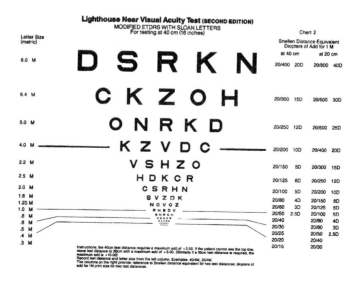

FIGURE 1-2 The ETDRS single-letter chart.

LIGHTHOUSE "CONTINUOUS TEXT" CARD FOR ADULTS
FOR NEAR VISION
LINE INCREMENTS IN LogMAR UNITS

	SNELLEN EQUIVALENT	METR PRINT SIZE

The bee stings.

20/400   8.0M

Butterflies taste with their hind feet.

20/320   6.4M

Ducks will lay eggs only in the morning.

20/250   5.0M

It is impossible to sneeze and keep one's eyes open.

20/200   4.0M

THIS CARD IS CALIBRATED FOR USE AT 40 CM (16 IN.) WITH CUSTOMARY READING CORRECTION IF NEEDED.

LIGHTHOUSE   LOW VISION PRODUCTS 36-02 NORTHERN BLVD., LONG ISLAND CITY, N.Y. 11101

©1989
CAT. NO. C 202

FIGURE 1-3 Lighthouse continuous text card.

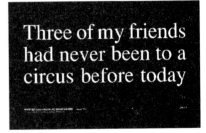

Three of my friends
had never been to a
circus before today

Three of my friends
had never been to a
circus before today

FIGURE 1-4 MNREAD acuity charts.

Legge added a new dimension when he introduced the MNREAD Low Vision Acuity Charts as a practical test for reading performance. There are 30 8.5 × 11 inch cards (Fig. 1-4) that contain a single sentence printed in black-on-white on one side and white-on-black on the other. The sentences are matched for visual layout and linguistic properties. A second set of MNREAD acuity charts (Fig. 1-5) ranges from 1.3 logMAR (20/400) to –0.5 logMAR (20/6.3) in 0.1 logMAR increments when viewed at 40 cm (16 inches). The cards can be used to assess read-

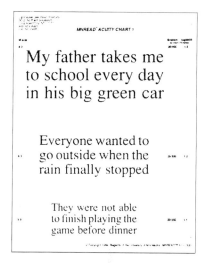 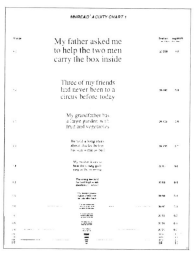

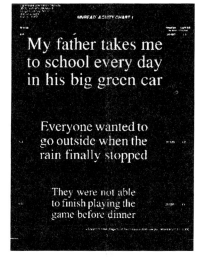 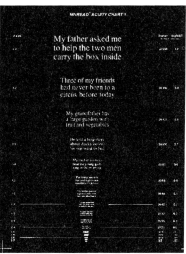

FIGURE 1-5 Standardized continuous text reading cards.

ing speed and acuity, and are also useful as tools in the low vision assessment and in prescribing magnifiers.

In 1983 further modifications were made, in keeping with the functional approach, when Faye and Rosenthal included a clinical contrast sensitivity function (CSF) test (Fig. 1-6) to the low vision evaluation. They suggested that contrast sensitivity testing was integral to the management of low vision patients and could be used to predict the need for higher magnification or increased illumination.

They also recommended that CSF be included in the initial and subsequent evaluations. Shortly thereafter other low vision clinicians began

VISION CONTRAST TEST SYSTEM

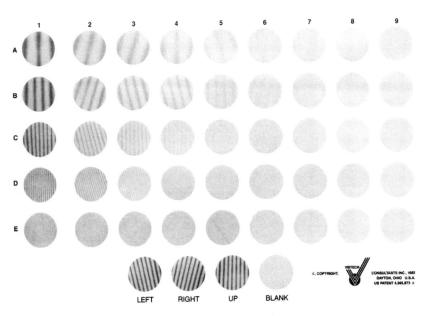

FIGURE 1-6 The clinical contrast sensitivity function test.

CLINICAL PEARL

Faye and Rosenthal have suggested that contrast sensitivity testing is integral to the management of low vision patients and can be used to predict the need for higher magnification or increased illumination.

to develop and include their own contrast sensitivity tests as part of the low vision battery. Bailey added a high-low vision contrast sensitivity test for adults, and along with the Mr. Happy pediatric CSF test, additional clinical contrast sensitivity tests were developed by Pelli et al.,[15] Johnson,[16] and Hyvarinen (Fig. 1-7). Faye has also recommended including the brightness acuity test in the low vision battery when one of the presenting complaints is glare.

CLINICAL PEARL

Faye has also recommended including the brightness acuity test in the low vision battery when one of the presenting complaints is glare.

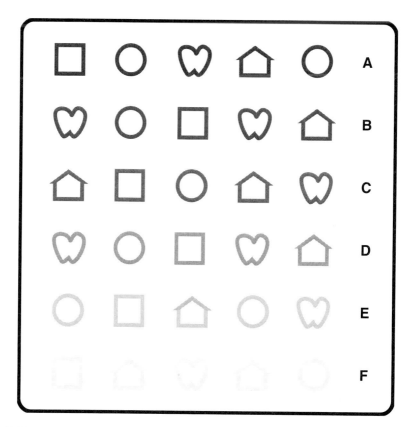

FIGURE 1-7 The clinical contrast sensitivity function test.

Feinbloom's Case History

Dr. William Feinbloom revolutionized history taking in low vision care by emphasizing the importance of assessing the impact of vision loss on the performance of daily activities. Low vision clinicians have seen the value of taking more specialized clinical histories since Feinbloom[17] made recommendations in 1935. The following overview of Dr. Feinbloom's history gives a historical perspective and rationale for many of the questions that are included in present-day low vision histories.

Feinbloom's suggestions for a complete case history included age of onset, duration of the subnormal visual condition, change in vision during the past 5 years, 2 years, and 6 months, diagnosis and prognosis by other practitioners, and whether the patient could get about unescorted. This, in fact, was the first indication of the importance of visual field and was a precursor to the inclusion of a section on questions regarding mobility.

Feinbloom went on to incorporate questions on whether the patient could see better in daylight or at night and when the patient had last been to the movies ("moving pictures"). The former question, of course, revolved around peripheral and/or central retinal function and, again, had relevance in the patient's mobility under varying conditions of illumination. The latter related to the effect of relative distance magnification. In fact, Dr. Feinbloom noted that "moving pictures" present objects magnified 2½ to 3 times their normal size and individuals no longer attending movies perhaps lose at least that amount of vision.

Other questions included when a patient had last read the newspaper, whether the patient could read large headlines, subheadlines, or small print, and whether the patient was still using separate distance and reading glasses. Also asked were questions on whether the patient saw better with an opera glass or magnifier and which eye functioned better. Finally, whether the patient could recognize red, blue, and green colors was elicited.

However, the most important questions that Dr. Feinbloom included related to what the patient *wanted* to do. For example, he asked about playing cards, writing brief letters, and seeing food on the table. He also stated that it was advisable not to spend too long taking the case history, noting that it "usually led to no satisfactory results." So we have the early beginnings of an extensive case history taking, by one individual, that addressed the primary objectives of the patient. The majority of clinicians up to that time were taking a history but neglecting to relate their findings to the patient's objectives.

Comprehensive Case History

The functional low vision evaluation can therefore be thought of as a series of clues that are used to solve the low vision patient–management puzzle. It begins with a comprehensive case history and concludes with a series of options that may include the prescription of low vision optical or nonoptical devices, referral to the primary care practitioner, or intervention by other rehabilitation professionals (i.e., professionals specializing in orientation and mobility, social services, or techniques of daily living).

CLINICAL PEARL

The functional low vision evaluation can be thought of as a series of clues that are used to solve the low vision patient–management puzzle.

The Lighthouse Low Vision Examination Form Intake History (Appendix) has been in development for over 20 years and will continue to evolve along with changes in the management of low vision patients. What has changed is that the initial intake is done by a social worker over the telephone before the low vision evaluation. The clinician then takes a more extensive ocular and medical history (when the patient arrives for evaluation) and reviews any areas that are major concerns.

The case history and low vision examination essentially provide clues to solving the larger puzzle of achieving successful outcomes for the low vision patient. The Lighthouse Low Vision Examination form includes an extensive ocular and medical history. Questions in the ocular history may relate to surgeries, laser or other treatments, and medications. Management of conditions (e.g., cataract, glaucoma, macular degeneration, diabetic retinopathy) has undergone major changes in the past 25 years, leading to new questions that the clinician must ask. For example, surgical treatment of cataract in the 1950s and 60s often resulted in large keyhole pupils that, in turn, led to symptoms of glare. Absorptive lenses and cosmetic contact lenses were often prescribed to eliminate the glare. Today individuals with keyhole pupils are rarely seen by the low vision clinician, but clinicians must be aware of any medical advances in ocular surgery that might result in unforeseen visual complaints.

CLINICAL PEARL

Clinicians must be aware of any medical advances in ocular surgery that might result in unforeseen visual complaints.

For example, if laser treatment has been performed for macular degeneration or diabetic retinopathy, questions about glare and mobility at night should be included with the standard inquiries about the number and frequency of treatments in each eye. Individuals receiving miotics should be questioned as to glare, especially if there are existing lens changes. Such questioning seeks to relate the pathology to visual function, as put forth by Faye.[4]

CLINICAL PEARL

Questions should be insightful and relevant to the existing eye condition.

The intake history also includes a section concerned with the living situation. Questions in this section should be directed toward employment status and social activities. Other concerns that need to be addressed are who will accompany the patient and in what language the examination will be conducted. The most comprehensive area in the intake history is the task analysis. This includes subsections on traveling, distance viewing, activities of daily living, near tasks, lighting considerations, and job/school-related tasks—all of which are important indicators of the person's mobility and orientation, need for optical treatment, daily living techniques, or job training to solve a stated problem. Thorough investigation of the tasks, plus emphasis on the patient's own assessments of his or her ability to complete them, makes this the most extensive part of the intake history.

The tests of visual function will be explored throughout the remainder of this book. Those that should be included in the initial low vision evaluation are a measurement of habitual and corrected incoming visual acuities at distance and near, an assessment of central visual field, contrast sensitivity, and color vision, and an analysis of visual field and brightness acuity when indicated. Follow-up examinations should also include visual acuity, Amsler grid, and contrast sensitivity.

Following is a suggested sequential low vision examination procedure. It comes after the extensive case history just outlined and includes charts for functional evaluation. (The *numbers* below correspond to those in the Lighthouse catalog, and items marked with an *asterisk* are presently used in the Lighthouse examination.)

1. Visual acuity
   a. Distance charts
      (1) Adult
         (a) ETDRS rear-illuminated standardized Ferris-Bailey chart* (acuity range 4/4 [20/20] to 1/40 [20/800])—recommended for clinical research
         (b) Letter—*C105, *C110, *C115
         (c) Number—*C102
         (d) Chart illuminator stand—*L225 (and illuminator—*L220)
      (2) Child
         (a) LH symbol chart—*C315
         (b) LH individual symbols (pediatric)—*C326
         (c) LH flip symbols—*C320 or *C321
         (d) Lighthouse flash card (house, apple, umbrella)—C150
         (e) Three-dimensional LH set—*C350
      (3) Designs for Vision: Revised number chart (still preferred by many clinicians)*; used to measure visual acuities as low as 20/14,000
   b. Initial test distance
      (1) ETDRS
         (a) Start at 2M
         (b) Switch to 1M when top line cannot be seen

(c) Use 4M with good visual acuity when visual field is the primary problem

  (2) Designs for Vision

    (a) Initially start at 10 feet or 2 M

    (b) Move in toward the patient when the chart cannot be seen

  c. Sequences of presentation

    (1) Visual acuity with correction OU/OD/OS

    (2) Visual acuity without correction OU/OD/OS

    (3) NOTE: Do not take an uncorrected distance acuity with a high refractive error

  d. The preferred recording of distance visual acuity for low vision patients is M notation (Chapter 2).

  e. Additional procedures in taking a distance acuity

    (1) Pinhole (or multiple pinhole when indicated)

    (2) Viewing eccentrically (left, right, up, down, oblique) to see if there is a preferred retinal locus

    (3) Occlusion (low vision patients often view eccentrically; to prevent "peeking," be sure that the occluder covers the entire eye

  f. Illumination

    (1) ETDRS: Turn illumination off to see if visual acuity improves

    (2) Designs for Vision: Vary illumination

    (3) Johnson[16] (p. 406) suggestion: Distance visual acuity at high (>1000 lux) and low (<30 lux) luminance when acuity is less than normal and ametropia is not suspected as the cause of reduction.

  g. Use of correction(s): Measure visual acuity only with current distance, near (bifocal), and sun prescriptions; eliminate old prescriptions not being worn

2. Glasses and low vision devices

  a. Note tints on the glasses

  b. Note age of the prescriptions

  c. List current low vision devices

    (1) Spectacles

    (2) Hand magnifiers (neutralize with loose lenses)

    (3) Stand magnifiers

    (4) Telescopes

    (5) Absorptive lenses

3. Incoming assessment of near visual acuity

  a. Chart

    (1) Lighthouse game card—*C191

    (2) Lighthouse flash card tests—C150

  b. Illumination: 60-watt bulb 1 foot from the page

  c. Habitual working distance: NOTE (in centimeters)

4. Gross external evaluation: Do not shine bright lights for any length of time into the eye at this point in the examination
   a. Note position of the eyes
   b. Note the pupils
      (1) Size
      (2) Reaction to light
      (3) Appearance
      (4) Position
      (5) Reflexes
   c. Note the irises
      (1) Transillumination
      (2) Iridectomies
   d. Note the corneas
      (1) Opacities
      (2) Size
      (3) Density
      (4) Position
   e. Note the lenses
      (1) Opacities
         (a) Nuclear
         (b) Anterior
         (c) Posterior
         (d) Mixed
      (2) Position (IOL)
   f. Note the motility
      (1) Nystagmus
      (2) Strabismus
      (3) Restrictions
5. Keratometry
   a. Initial evaluation
   b. Especially if keratoconus is suspected
   c. Albinism
   d. Corneal involvement
   e. High cylinders
6. Retinoscopy
   a. Trial frame
   b. Over refraction using a Halberg-type clip-on
      (1) High refractive error
      (2) Patient unable to tolerate weight of the trial frame
   c. Avoid use of the phoropter (especially with eccentric viewing and a high refractive error)
   d. Poor retinal reflex
      (1) Start with the patient's previous prescription
      (2) Redo retinoscopy off axis
      (3) Radical retinoscopy—i.e., move toward the patient to see if there is a retinal reflex
      (4) Use a loose high-power lens (e.g., ± 4.00 or ± 8.00)

7. Subjective
   a. Note the patient's response
      (1) Significant improvement
      (2) Somewhat better
      (3) Minimal improvement
      (4) No improvement
   b. Just noticeable difference (JND) lens to use in refining the sphere: Divide the numerator of the Snellen fraction/denominator by 2; examples of lenses to use are
      (1) Visual acuity 2M—equivalent VA 20/200 JND ± 1.00
      (2) Visual acuity 4M—equivalent VA 20/400 JND ± 2.00
      (3) Visual acuity 8M—equivalent VA 20/800 JND ± 4.00
   c. Hand-held Jackson cross cylinder: Generally used in powers of ± 0.50, *0.75, *1.00
   d. Refining cylinder
      (1) Exaggerated technique for power
      (2) Rotation of cylinder for axis
8. Prediction of the near add
   a. Chart
      (1) adults—Lighthouse near visual acuity card for adults—*C170
      (2) pediatric—LH symbols—*C330 (single symbols), C335 (multiple symbols)
   b. To determine single letter acuity, hold the card at 40 cm with a +2.50 add (for absolute presbyopes) over the best distance correction; if the patient cannot read the 8M (top line of chart), (see 9.c)
      (1) 4M requires a +10 D add over the distance correction
         (a) Distance correction is plano—starting lens is +10 D
         (b) Distance lens is +6.00—starting lens is +16.00 D
         (c) Distance correction is –4.50 = –3.50 × 90—starting lens is +5.50 = –3.50 × 90
      (2) 8M requires a +20 D add over the distance correction
      (3) Predicted add is the starting lens for selection of spectacles and a hand or stand magnifier
   c. Repeat the test at 20 cm with a +5.00 add over the best distance refraction when the top line of the ETDRS chart cannot be read
      (1) 10M requires a 25 D add over the best distance correction
      (2) 16M requires a 40 D add over the best distance correction
   d. Continuous text acuity
      (1) Lighthouse continuous text card for adults—*C202
      (2) Children's Lighthouse continuous text chart—*C212
      (3) Lighthouse continuous text card in Spanish
      (4) Hoeft near reading card
      (5) MNREAD acuity charts
         (a) White on black—C400, C410
         (b) Black on white—C405, C415

(6) MNREAD low vision reading cards—C420 (three cards)
  (a) Continuous text series, large print
  (b) Continuous text series, small paragraphs
  (c) Continuous text, white on black
(7) Designs for Vision near reading cards
  (a) English
  (b) Spanish
  (c) Hebrew
  (d) Arabic
(8) University of North Carolina near vision test with short words and single optotypes in meter, Jaeger, and point print (included is a typoscope)—C185
e. Assessing reading speed
  (1) MNREAD low vision reading cards—C420 (three cards)
    (a) Continuous text series, large print
    (b) Continuous text series, small paragraphs
    (c) Continuous text, white on black

9. Amsler grid
  a. Chart
    (1) No. 1: White letters on a black background
    (2) No. 2: For poor fixation (with diagonals included)
  b. Test distance—33 cm
  c. Correction—+3.00 over the best distance correction
  d. Sequence—OU, OD, OS (note that OU is performed first)
  e. Illumination—60 W, 1 foot from the page
  f. Recording of scotoma(s)
    (1) Position
    (2) Density
    (3) Size
    (4) Appearance of horizontal and vertical lines (note any waviness)
    (5) Size of the boxes
    (6) Note the contrast of the grid independently and compare it with that for the other eye

10. Contrast sensitivity function (distance charts)
  a. Vision contrast test system—*C225
    (1) Test distance: 1 meter
    (2) Sequence: OD, OS, OU
    (3) Record on a low vision recording sheet findings from (a) and (b)
  b. Additional contrast sensitivity tests used in low vision
    (1) Vector vision
    (2) Pelli-Robson—letter triplet chart
    (3) Bailey
      (a) Adult high/low
      (b) Pediatric Mr. Happy

       (4) Lea symbols—C345, C346

       (5) Johnston—high/low

    c. Illumination

       (1) Use the recommended light meter for Vistech charts

       (2) Check the manufacturer's specifications for all other charts

11. Color vision (see Chapters 7 and 8)

    a. Adults

       (1) D-15 series

          (a) Standard size

          (b) Large

          (c) Lanthony desaturated test

          (d) Adams desaturated

       (2) Color plates

          (a) AO-HRR (American Optical–Hardy-Rand-Rittler) test

          (b) Ishihara's test for color blindness

          (c) Pseudoisochromatic plates for acquired color vision defects

    b. Pediatric

          (a) LH (large) quantitative color vision test

          (b) Use similar to that for D-15

          (c) Matching test

    c. Illumination: Generally illuminant C

12. Visual fields (Chapter 6)

    a. Goldmann type

    b. Automated

    c. Tangent screen

13. Prescription for standard spectacle correction

    a. Distance

    b. Near

    c. Intermediate

    d. Bifocal

    e. Trifocal

    f. Hold off till the next visit

14. Presentation of low vision devices: It is important to remember the power of the initial starting lens is determined by the predicted add

    a. Spectacles

       (1) Available systems

          (a) Half-eye with prism

          (b) Full field

          (c) Doublet/telephoto

       (2) Recommendations for the other eye

          (a) Plano

          (b) Alternate

          (c) Occlude

          (d) Frost

   b. Hand magnifiers
     (1) Nonilluminated
     (2) Illuminated
   c. Stand magnifiers
     (1) Nonilluminated
     (2) Illuminated
   d. Telescopic lenses
     (1) Hand held
     (2) Spectacle mounted
       (a) Bioptic
         (i) Galilean/Keplerian
         (ii) Standard/micro (Clearview)
       (b) Full diameter
         (i) Galilean/Keplerian
       (c) Reading
         (i) Galilean/Keplerian
       (d) Across-the-bridge (VES)
       (e) Behind-the-lens
     (3) Use of the Hoeft training shield
   e. Absorptive lenses
     (1) NoIR
       (a) Wraparound
       (b) Clip-on
     (2) Corning Photochromatic Filter
       (a) clip-on—450, 511, 527, 527DN, 550, 550XD
       (b) prescriptive
     (3) Polaroid
     (4) Slip-behind
     (5) Clip-on
     (6) Dyed
     (7) Visor
   f. Nonoptical/accessory devices
   g. Illumination control/nonoptical devices/other
     (1) Recommendations
       (a) Bright
       (b) Moderate
       (c) Dim
       (d) Avoid glare
     (2) Lamps
       (a) Incandescent
       (b) Halogen
       (c) Neodymium
     (3) Bulb
     (4) Typoscope
     (5) Amber filter paper
     (6) Felt-tip pen

        (7) Writing guide
        (8) Signature guide
        (9) Large print
        (10) Large-print check
        (11) Lap desk
        (12) Phone aid
        (13) In-touch radio
        (14) Talking book
        (15) Other
      h. Closed-circuit TV
        (1) Note the magnification necessary
        (2) Preference on polarity
15. Assessment/plan
    a. Were the patient's objectives met?
16. Counseling provided
    a. Diagnostic results/impressions, including vision status
    b. Instructions for management/treatment
    c. Treatment optics
      (1) advantages/disadvantages of the different magnifiers
      (2) lighting
      (3) other services/resources (e.g., slit lamp evaluation)
    d. Patient and family education
      (1) eye condition
    e. Prognosis
    f. Risk factor reduction
17. Time spent on counseling/education (minutes and/or percent of exam)
18. Slit lamp evaluation
19. Supplementary testing procedures
    a. Electrodiagnostics
      (1) Visual evoked potential (VEP)
      (2) Electroretinogram (ERG)
    b. Ultrasound
      (1) A-scan
      (2) B-scan
    c. Dark adaptometry
    d. Magnetic resonance imaging (MRI)
    e. Computed tomography (CT)
20. Additional referral services
    a. Social
    b. Orientation/mobility
    c. Career/technology
    d. Rehabilitation—training for activities of daily living
21. Is the patient legally blind?
    a. Registered with the CBVH?
    b. Should the patient be registered?

22. Visual impairment descriptor code
23. Eye diagnosis
    a. Primary
    b. Secondary

References

1. Mehr E, Freid A: *Low vision care*, Chicago, 1975, Professional Press, pp 13-24, 81-104.
2. Faye E: *The low vision patient*, New York, 1970, Grune & Stratton.
3. Newman J: *A guide to the care of low vision patients*, St. Louis, 1974, American Optometric Association.
4. Faye E: *Clinical low vision*, ed 2, Boston, 1984, Little Brown.
5. Rosenthal B, Cole RG: *A structured approach to low vision care*, Philadelphia, 1991, JB Lippincott, Vol 3, no. 3.
6. Cole RG, Rosenthal B: *Patient and practice management in low vision*, Philadelphia, 1992, JB Lippincott, Vol 4, no. 1.
7. Freeman PB, Jose RT: *The art and practice of low vision*, Stoneham, Mass, 1991, Butterworth-Heinemann.
8. Nowakowski R: *Primary low vision care*, Norwalk, 1994, Appleton & Lange.
9. Bailey IL, Lovie SJE: New design principles for visual acuity letter chart, *Am J Optom Physiol Opt* 53:740-745, 1976.
10. Bailey IL, Lovie SJE: The design and use of a new near vision chart, *Am J Optom Physiol Opt* 57:378-388, 1980.
11. Ferris FL 3d, Kassoff A, Bresnick GH, Bailey I: New visual acuity charts for clinical research, *Am J Ophthalmol* 94:91-96, 1982.
12. Bailey IL: A call for the elimination of the Jaeger and reduced Snellen notations, *Optom Month* 69:676-679, 1978.
13. Bailey I: Specification of nearpoint performance, *Optom Month* 69:895-898, 1978.
14. Faye E, Rosenthal BP, Hood C, Seidman K: *The New York Lighthouse low vision continuing education curriculum*, New York, 1984, The Lighthouse.
15. Pelli DG, Robson JG, Wilkins AJ: The design of a new letter chart for measurement of contrast sensitivity, *Clin Vis Sci* 3:187-199, 1988.
16. Johnston AW: Making sense of the M, N, and logMAR systems of specifying visual acuity. In Rosenthal B, Cole RG: *A structured approach to low vision care*, Philadelphia, 1991, JB Lippincott, Vol 3, no. 3.
17. Feinbloom W: Introduction to the principle and practice of subnormal correction, *J Am Optom Assoc* 6:13-18, 1935.

Appendix—Lighthouse low vision examination form intake history

(Use label or complete box below)

Date ____ / ____ / ____
Start time _____

Name _____ Case no. _____	
Street _____ Apt ____ Phone (___) _____ SS no. ____ / ____ / ____	
City _____ State ____ Zip_____ Age ____ DOB ____ / ____ / ____	

Referred by: _____ Eye doctor (same) _____
Do you wish us to send a report to your doctor: Y   N

Previous low vision care: Y   N   If Yes, when and where?_____
If No, does the person understand why he/she is coming in (i.e., purpose of exam)?   Y   N
Previous low vision devices: Y   N   From whom, if different from above? _____

Reported   OD_____   OS_____
diagnoses   _____   _____

OCULAR HISTORY (surgeries, laser or other treatments, eye medications) _____
_____
_____
_____
_____
_____

Last eye exam _____ Onset _____ Better eye   **R   L   Unsure**

Has your vision changed significantly in the past month?   **Y   N**
Since your last opthalmological exam?   **Y   N**
Does your vision fluctuate from day to day?   **Y   N**   How is it today? _____

GENERAL HEALTH HISTORY (circle positive findings and reference below by number)
Medical conditions (e.g., [1] diabetes, [2] hypertension, [3] heart disease, [4] arthritis,
   [5] Parkinson's, [6] thyroid, [7] allergies, [8] other; please list medications by condition)
_____
_____
_____
_____
_____

Hearing loss   **Y   N**   If yes, specify_____ Hearing aid?   **Y   N**

LIVING SITUATION (alone, spouse, children, nursing home, aide, etc.) _____
_____

Employment status
___Retired   ___Employed/Full Time   ___Unemployed/Seeking Employment
___On leave   ___Employed/Part Time   ___Unemployed/Not Seeking Employment
___Homemaker

Reason for status or job description _____
_____ Is your job in jeopardy? **Y   N   N/A**
Have you considered retiring/resigning because of your vision? **Y   N   N/A**

Social activities (senior ctr, church, etc.)_____

Other limitations (difficulty walking, tremors, etc.)_____

Sponsored CBVH? **Y N**   CBVH no.   RSE? **Y N**   ASP? **Y N**   Other _____

Agency/Counselor _____ Previous Other Rehab _____

Adaptive/Mobility equipment _____

Who will accompany patient to the exam? _____ Phone (___)_____

Speaks English?   **Y N**   If not, can patient bring interpreter?   **Y N**

Primary language (if not English) _____

TASK ANALYSIS Circle each as   N/A, Not applicable   N, No problem
       M, Mild problem   Y, Major problem   O, Patient objective

a. Traveling: Do you go out alone?   Y   N   **Chief complaint/**
            (if no, skip to b)   **misses most**

"Do you have difficulty"
1. Traveling locally alone?   N/A   N   M   Y   O
2. Traveling far alone?   N/A   N   M   Y   O   **Additional history**
3. Seeing to drive a car?   N/A   N   M   Y   O   (reference by no./letter)
4. Seeing traffic lights?   N/A   N   M   Y   O   (for doctor's use **only**)
5. Seeing street signs?   N/A   N   M   Y   O
6. Crossing streets?   N/A   N   M   Y   O

b. Distance viewing

"Do you have difficulty"
7. Getting around
    people/objects?   N/A   N   M   Y   O
8. Seeing curbs and stairs?   N/A   N   M   Y   O
9. Walking without falling?   N/A   N   M   Y   O
10. Seeing faces?   N/A   N   M   Y   O
11. Seeing the TV? (distance___)   N/A   N   M   Y   O
12. Seeing at the theater?   N/A   N   M   Y   O

c. Daily living activities

"Do you have difficulty"
13. Doing your housework?   N/A   N   M   Y   O
14. Seeing to cook?   N/A   N   M   Y   O
15. Seeing stove dials?   N/A   N   M   Y   O
16. Seeing flame on stove?   N/A   N   M   Y   O
17. Seeing food on your plate?   N/A   N   M   Y   O
18. Seeing a phone/
     using a phone?   N/A   N   M   Y   O
19. Seeing to groom yourself   N/A   N   M   Y   O

d. Near tasks

"Do you have difficulty"

<table>
<tr><td>20. Reading headlines?
(if yes, skip to 27)</td><td>N/A</td><td>N</td><td>M</td><td>Y</td><td>O</td></tr>
<tr><td>21. Reading regular-print books?</td><td>N/A</td><td>N</td><td>M</td><td>Y</td><td>O</td></tr>
<tr><td>22. Reading newsprint/
small print?</td><td>N/A</td><td>N</td><td>M</td><td>Y</td><td>O</td></tr>
<tr><td>23. Seeing prices/labels?</td><td>N/A</td><td>N</td><td>M</td><td>Y</td><td>O</td></tr>
<tr><td>24. Reading your mail/bills?</td><td>N/A</td><td>N</td><td>M</td><td>Y</td><td>O</td></tr>
<tr><td>25. Reading handwritten
material?</td><td>N/A</td><td>N</td><td>M</td><td>Y</td><td>O</td></tr>
<tr><td>26. Writing/signing name
(on checks, etc.)?</td><td>N/A</td><td>N</td><td>M</td><td>Y</td><td>O</td></tr>
<tr><td>27. Seeing colors?</td><td>N/A</td><td>N</td><td>M</td><td>Y</td><td>O</td></tr>
<tr><td>28. Filling a syringe (diabetics)?</td><td>N/A</td><td>N</td><td>M</td><td>Y</td><td>O</td></tr>
<tr><td>29. Seeing your meds/labels?</td><td>N/A</td><td>N</td><td>M</td><td>Y</td><td>O</td></tr>
<tr><td>30. Seeing to sew/knit/crochet?</td><td>N/A</td><td>N</td><td>M</td><td>Y</td><td>O</td></tr>
<tr><td>31. Seeing playing cards?</td><td>N/A</td><td>N</td><td>M</td><td>Y</td><td>O</td></tr>
</table>

Other _____

e. Lighting considerations

"Do you have problems"

<table>
<tr><td>32. Tolerating the sun well?</td><td>N/A</td><td>N</td><td>M</td><td>Y</td><td>O</td></tr>
<tr><td>33. On cloudy/rainy days?</td><td>N/A</td><td>N</td><td>M</td><td>Y</td><td>O</td></tr>
<tr><td>34. Seeing in dim light?</td><td>N/A</td><td>N</td><td>M</td><td>Y</td><td>O</td></tr>
<tr><td>35. Going from bright to
dim light?</td><td>N/A</td><td>N</td><td>M</td><td>Y</td><td>O</td></tr>
<tr><td>36. Do you wear sunglasses?</td><td>N/A</td><td>N</td><td>M</td><td>Y</td><td>O</td></tr>
<tr><td>37. Are the sunglasses effective?</td><td>N/A</td><td>N</td><td>M</td><td>Y</td><td>O</td></tr>
<tr><td>38. Does a bright light help you?</td><td>N/A</td><td>N</td><td>M</td><td>Y</td><td>O</td></tr>
</table>

Preferred light source: (circle)
Incandescent   Fluorescent   Hi-Intensity   Other _____

f. Job/School related tasks N/A

(Complete only if employment status on p. 1 indicates)

"Do you have difficulty"

<table>
<tr><td>39. Using a computer?</td><td>N/A</td><td>N</td><td>M</td><td>Y</td><td>O</td></tr>
<tr><td>40. Using tools/equipment?</td><td>N/A</td><td>N</td><td>M</td><td>Y</td><td>O</td></tr>
<tr><td>41. Reading instruments/
indicators?</td><td>N/A</td><td>N</td><td>M</td><td>Y</td><td>O</td></tr>
<tr><td>42. Moving within work site/
school?</td><td>N/A</td><td>N</td><td>M</td><td>Y</td><td>O</td></tr>
<tr><td>43. Seeing the blackboard
in class?</td><td>N/A</td><td>N</td><td>M</td><td>Y</td><td>O</td></tr>
</table>

Task analysis completed by _____
(Initials)

Patient's name _____
(or attach label here)

Additional history
(reference by no./letter)
(for doctor's use **only**)

_____
_____
_____
_____
_____
_____
_____
_____
_____
_____
_____
_____
_____
_____
_____
_____
_____
_____
_____
_____
_____
_____
_____
_____
_____
_____
_____
_____

Major objectives _____
_____

General description
of patient _____
_____
_____

Patient attitude (e.g.,
realistic, depressed, anxious)
_____
_____

Eye report/Intake reviewed
(Doctor's initials) _____

VISUAL ACUITY

a. Vsc   OD _____ OS _____ OU _____ Pinhole: OD _____ OS _____

b. Vcc   Present status: No Rx ___ SV ___ BF _____ Prog ___ CLs ___ Other _____

(1) Distance Rx   OD _____ <u>V</u>A: OD _____

   Age of Rx ____

         OU _____

   Tint _____ OS _____ OS _____

   Reading Rx   OD _____ OD _____

   Age of Rx ____

         OU _____

       OS _____ OS _____

(2) Distance Rx   OD _____ OD _____

   Age of Rx ____

         OU _____

   Tint _____ OS _____ OS _____

   Reading Rx   OD _____ OD _____

   Age of Rx ____

         OU _____

       OS _____ OS _____

c. Current stock of low vision devices (spectacles/HMs/SMs/TSs/Sunwear)

   ____ Did not bring to exam

   List/VA _____

   _____

   _____

Gross external abnormalities (details on p. 000) _____

REFRACTIVE EVALUATION Cycloplegic **Y N** Trial Frame ___ Halberg clip-ons ___

Keratometry   OD _____ OS _____

Retinoscopy   OD _____ OS _____

Subjective   OD _____ VA ___ OS _____ VA ___

Patient's response to subjective:

  Significant improvement/Some improvement/Minimal improvement/No improvement

NEAR VISUAL ACUITY TEST

  Add used: +2.50 _____ Other _____ Test distance: 40 cm _____ Other _____

OD ___ OS ___ OU ___ Predicted add for 1.0 m _____   Test used SL/no./SW/CT

FUNCTIONAL TESTING   Amsler grids

  OU   OD   OS

BAT	OD	OS
Off		
Low		
Med		
Hi		

Contrast sensitivity 1 Meter _____   Near _____   (low normal value in [])

OD   Row A ___ [4]   Row B ___ [5]   Row C ___ [4]   Row D ___ [5]   Row E ___ [5]

OS   Row A ___ [4]   Row B ___ [5]   Row C ___ [4]   Row D ___ [5]   Row E ___ [5]

OU   Row A ___ [4]   Row B ___ [5]   Row C ___ [4]   Row D ___ [5]   Row E ___ [5]

Color testing _____ Test used _____ Results OD _____ OS _____

Other visual field testing (confrontations, Goldmann VF, tangent screen) _____

TRIAL OF LOW VISION DEVICES: Review of goals _____

Base Rx (for testing): Patient's own, refraction, other (indicate below)

Distance: OD _____   Near   OD _____
                                    (nonstock):
              OS _____   OS _____

Dominant eye: OD   OS   Better functional Eye: OD   OS   OU

Spectacles (AO, Aolites; CI, Clear Image; FF, full field; 1/2, half eye; Other)
Better with Typoscope? **Y   N**

Power/Type	Eye(s)	SW VA	CT VA	Dist.	Comments	Try*
		M				
		M				
		M				
		M				

Hand magnifiers (B & L, Bausch & Lomb; C, Coil; E = Eschenbach; S = Selsi; Other)

Power/Brand/Type/IL	Eye(s)	SW VA	CT VA	Dist.	Comments/Rx used	Try*
		M				
		M				
		M				
		M				

Stand magnifiers (B & L, Bausch & Lomb; C, Coil; E, Eschenbach; P, Peak; S, Selsi; Other)

Power/Brand/Type/IL	Eye(s)	SW VA	CT VA	Dist.	Comments/Rx used	Try*
		M				
		M				
		M				
		M				

Telescopes (E, Eschenbach; LH, Lighthouse; S, Selsi; B, Beecher; Other)

Power/Type	Eye(s)	Dist VA	NearVA	Dist.	Comments	Try*
		M				
		M				
		M				

*Try: Indicate recommendations as (L) loaner or (D) dispense; prioritize by number, if appropriate.

For spectacles: Other eye   Alternate   Plano   Occlude   Frost

Illumination control/nonoptical devices/Other:
Lamps _____   Felt-tip pens _____   Large print _____   Phone aids _____
Bulbs _____   Bold line paper _____   LP check _____   In-touch radio _____
Typoscope _____   Writing guide _____   Check guide _____   Talking books _____
Amber filter _____   Signature guide _____   Lap desk _____   Other _____

NOTES _____
_____
_____
_____

OTHER RECOMMENDATIONS FOR TRAINING/PRESCRIBING/DEMONSTRATING

New spectacle Rx? (details on dispensing form) **Y   N**
Type: Dist   Near   Intermediate   Bifocal

Hold Rx until RV/FU _____   Trifocal   Other _____

Illumination Near Bright Moderate Dim Avoid glare Comment _____

Sunwear Demo: **Y   N** UV Shield __ Other Noir __ CPF __ Visor __ Other _____

Specific Color(s) to be tested _____

CCTV demo: **Y   N** _____ Magnification _____ Working distance _____

Training needed: Eccentric viewing   Distance   Near   Resists near WD with specs

TS spotting   Hemianopia   Scanning   Trouble focusing HM

ASSESSMENT/PLAN (were patient's goals/objectives met? Unusual devices or needs?)
_____
_____
_____
_____
_____
_____
_____
_____
_____
_____
_____

Counseling provided (indicate on checklist and provide specifics in space below,
   as necessary)
___ 1. Diagnostic results/Impressions (___ a. Vision status)
___ 2. Instructions for management/treatment
___ 3. Treatment options (___ a. Adv/Disadv of different magnifiers ___ b. Lighting
         ___ c. Other services/resources)
___ 4. Patient/Family education (___ a. Eye condition)
___ 5. Prognosis
___ 6. Risk factor reduction
_____
_____
_____
_____

Time spent on counseling/education (minutes and/or percent of exam)_____

REFERRALS
   O&M   ASP   Career services   Reg CBVH   Apply for services   Refer back to MD
   Other _____

Return for revisit with LV doctor? **Y   N**   When? _____
Is patient legally blind? **Y   N**   Registered CBVH? **Y   N**
If not, consents to be registered? **Y   N**

GENERAL OCULAR HEALTH ASSESSMENT (circle if normal, otherwise cross out and record findings)

Pupils: PERRL (–) MG _____

Motility, eye turn, nystagmus WNL _____

Lids (Ptosis, ectropion, etc.) clear_____

Cornea (opacities, size, etc.) clear _____

Iris (iridectomies, transillum, etc.) intact_____

Lens/IOL clear _____

Retina/Optic nerve (see diagram) _____

Other findings of note _____

_____

_____

IOP (If recorded) OD_____ OS_____ Time _____ DPA Instilled _____

Ophthalmoscopy   Anterior Segment
OD   OS   OD   OS

DIAGNOSES

Visual impairment descriptors	Primary eye medical diagnosis	Secondary eye medical diagnosis
OD _____	OD _____	OD _____
OS _____	OS _____	OS _____
Code _____	Code _____	Exam end time _____

OVERALL LEVEL OF COMPLEXITY OF CARE
(must agree with billing statement) 1 2 3 4 5
(was level selected based on counseling time? **Y**   **N**)

Clinician's signature _____   Date _____

Print name _____

LV EXAM

C H A P T E R

2

Visual Acuity and the Predicted Reading Add

Roy Gordon Cole

Key Terms

Low vision	Kestenbaum	Lighthouse
Snellen equivalent	Reciprocal of vision	Reading add
Predicting the add		

When beginning to work on near vision aids with the low vision patient, you need a starting point (the "predicted add"). An add should be presented that will allow the patient to function at or near the desired level, but not be too strong.

Various methods of predicting the reading add (i.e., the add power required to read standard or, in some cases, nonstandard print) are taught and have been discussed in the literature. This chapter will present a generalized basic concept for predicting the reading add and then will present and discuss the methods, showing how each is a variant of the basic concept.

Before proceeding, I would like to emphasize that no matter what method of predicting the add is used it gives you only a starting point. The patient must be evaluated with lenses in place, using his or her

Reprinted from *Journal of the American Optometric Association*, Volume 64, Number 1, January 1993. The article was originally titled "Predicting the Low Vision Reading Add."

desired reading material (not test charts), and modifications of lens power must be made until the patient's goals are reached.

CLINICAL PEARL

No matter what method of predicting the add is used, it gives you only a starting point.

A General "Basic Concept" for Predicting the Reading Add

The basic concept in predicting the needed add for the low vision patient is

$$\text{Predicted Add} = (\text{Magnification Ratio}) \times (\text{Reference Add})$$

The magnification required can be defined as the ratio of the present acuity level to the desired acuity level.

$$\text{Magnification Ratio} = \frac{\text{Present Acuity Level}}{\text{Desired Acuity Level}}$$

Both the present and the desired acuity level should be given as numbers representing the actual letter sizes (e.g., M values, Snellen equivalent denominator).[1] NOTE: the Snellen equivalent at near is sometimes referred to as the *reduced* Snellen equivalent. Thus, another way to write the magnification ratio is

$$\text{Magnification Ratio} = \frac{\text{Letter Size Can Read}}{\text{Letter Size Wants To Read}}$$

For this to be valid, both Snellen acuities must be referenced to the same distance. There must also be consistency in the units on the top and bottom of the magnification fraction.

The *reference add* (above and beyond the prescription giving the best-corrected distance acuity) is the add used when measuring the present acuity level (letter size can read). If the patient is tested at distance, the dioptric equivalent of the testing distance is used—e.g., at 4 m, a +0.25 D add is used. If the patient is tested at near, the power of the testing add is used.

Clinical Application of the Basic Concept

As an example of the application of this basic concept, consider an emmetropic patient who can read 20/200 Snellen (40M at 4 m) at far and who also reads 20/200 Snellen equivalent at 16 inches (4M at 0.4 m) through a +2.50 DS near prescription. He wants to read 1M (20/50 Snellen equivalent at 16 inches). What is the predicted add?

Calculating from the distance acuity

Using the metric acuities, the patient needs a reference add of +0.25 (4 m working distance). The magnification ratio is 40M/1M = 40×. Thus the predicted add is

$$(40)(0.25) = +10.00 \text{ D.}$$

The distance Snellen and near Snellen equivalent acuities (for "present acuity level" and "desired acuity level" respectively) cannot both be used in this ratio because they are not referenced to the same distance. A 20/200 letter at 20 feet has a different size than a 20/200 Snellen equivalent letter referenced to 16 inches (Fig. 2-1). For the basic concept to work with both distance and near Snellen acuities, a factor compensating for the physical size differences must be used. In this example a 20-foot letter is 15 times larger than a Snellen equivalent letter referenced to 16 inches:

$$(20 \text{ feet})/(16 \text{ inches}) = (240 \text{ inches})/(16 \text{ inches}) = 15 \ (\times \text{ Larger})$$

In other words, the near letter must be "enlarged" 15 times compared to the distance Snellen letter. This magnification ratio then becomes (200/50)(15) = 60×. At 20 feet (approximately 6 m, the distance at which the far 20/200 acuity is taken) the add used is 1/6 D. The predicted add is thus

$$(60)\left(\frac{1}{6}\right) = +10.00 \text{ D}$$

As can be seen, it is not easy to calculate a predicted add on the basis of a distance Snellen acuity and a near Snellen equivalent acuity; therefore this method is generally not used.

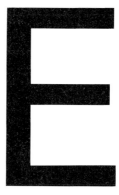

FIGURE 2-1 Comparison of distance and near 20/200 Snellen letters. The *E* on the left is a 20/200 Snellen equivalent designed to be used at 16 inches. The *E* on the right is 20/200 designed to be used at 20 feet. Note the physical difference in sizes.

The magnification ratio does work with near acuities, however, because if a near present acuity level is not given the assumption is made that the distance acuity is the same as the near acuity (e.g., 20/200 at far is translated to 20/200 Snellen equivalent at 16 inches). This is not a problem with metric acuities (the M system) because the M value represents the actual size of the letter, irrespective of the distance at which the test was done (Fig. 2-2).

Calculating from the near acuity

The patient is using a reference add of +2.50 D since the near present acuity level was taken at a standard viewing distance of 16 inches. The magnification ratio is 4× based on either the Snellen equivalent

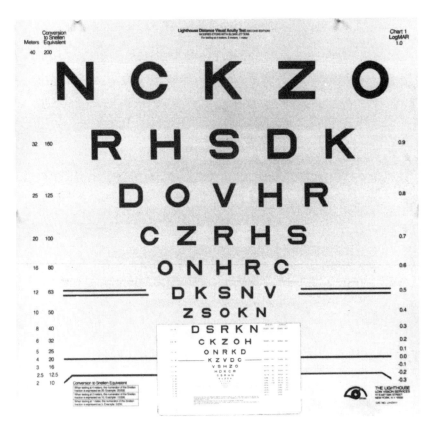

FIGURE 2-2 Comparison of distance and near metric acuity letters. The near chart is superimposed on the distance chart, over the letters that are the same size. Note that the near chart is the bottom of the distance chart (but extended to include the smaller letter sizes). A letter with a specific metric notation (1M, 4M, 8M) has the same physical size irrespective of which chart is used. (Courtesy Lighthouse Low Vision Products.)

denominators (200/50, both being referenced to 16 inches) or the M notations (4M/1M). The predicted add is thus

$$(4)(2.50) = +10.00 \text{ D}$$

The M System and Predicting the Add

An advantage of using the M system is that if your goal is 1M (a good approximation for standard newsprint) the predicted add is given by the product of the M value for the line read and the add used (reference add):

Predicted Add = (M Value Read) (Reference Add)

Note that the *M Value Read* actually represents a magnification ratio, with the denominator (desired acuity level) equal to 1. For example, a patient with a +2.50 DS distance refraction reads 5M print at a distance of about 12 inches with his old +6.00 DS reading lenses. His predicted add is thus

$$(5) (+3.50) = +17.50 \text{ D}$$

NOTE: The 5 represents the entering acuity read with these glasses, and the +3.50 is the add represented by the reading glasses (6.00 – 2.50). The entering acuity was at 12 inches, closer than would be expected with a +2.50 D add but appropriate for the +3.50 D add. The measurement of habitual entering near acuity test distance can give you valuable information. Other factors (e.g., pupil size, lens changes), however, can affect the habitual reading distance. We will not be considering these factors.

Three Commonly Used Methods to Predict the Add

Kestenbaum's Rule

Kestenbaum's Rule allows you to predict the add from the best-corrected distance acuity.

Method

To predict the add needed to read standard print, use the reciprocal of the best-corrected distance acuity. This number represents the dioptric value of the add.[2]

Example

A patient with 20/200 best-corrected acuity would be predicted to need a 200/20 = +10.00 D add. A patient with 20/400 acuity would need an add of 400/20 = +20.00 D. Generally the lower add (corresponding to better acuity) is used before both eyes as a starting point.

If distance acuity is measured in M notation, a fraction is still written and can be inverted. Thus the 20/200 patient would have an acuity of 4/40, or 2/20, etc. Inverting these acuities still gives the same predicted add of +10.00 D. Note that one advantage of testing with the M system at a 1-meter test distance is that the value of the line read in "M" notation also gives the predicted add in diopters. This is because the numerator of the acuity fraction is 1, which becomes the denominator when the fraction is inverted. Thus the patient reading 16M at a 1-meter test distance would be predicted to need a +16 D add.

Discussion

When several assumptions are applied to the basic concept, we can derive Kestenbaum's Rule. These assumptions are (1) distance and near acuities are comparable (i.e., you can assume the near acuity as being the same as the measured distance acuity), (2) the reference add is +2.50 D (i.e., the reference distance is 16 inches), and (3) the desired acuity level is 20/50 Snellen equivalent (at 16 inches) at near. The formula for the basic concept thus becomes

$$\text{Predicted Add} = \frac{\text{Distance Snellen Denominator}}{50} \times 2.50$$

Now, 2.50/50 is the same as 1/20, so the formula reduces to

$$\text{Predicted Add} = \frac{\text{Distance Snellen Denominator}}{20}$$

The right side of this equation is just the Snellen distance acuity inverted, which is the definition given for Kestenbaum's Rule. Note that the same reasoning can be applied when using the metric system.

Lighthouse Method

The Lighthouse Method allows you to read the predicted add directly from the near visual acuity chart.

Method

A +2.50 D add is placed over the patient's best spectacle correction, and the Lighthouse Near Visual Acuity Test Chart (Fig. 2-3) is held at 40 cm. (A +5.00 D add and a 20 cm working distance can be used if the patient's acuity is too poor for the weaker add.) The patient reads as far down the chart as possible. The predicted add for standard print (assumed to be 1M or 20/50 at 40 cm) is then read on the right-hand side of the chart opposite the last line read (Fig. 2-4). Be certain to look under the correct column: *at 40 cm* if a +2.50 D add is used, and *at 20 cm* if a +5.00 D add. The test is done monocularly, and generally the weaker of the two predicted adds (OD or OS) is the starting add.[3] It might be mentioned that this technique is based upon the Sloan method, the difference being

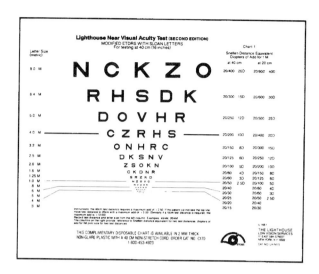

FIGURE 2-3 Lighthouse Near Visual Acuity Test Chart. (Courtesy Lighthouse Low Vision Products.)

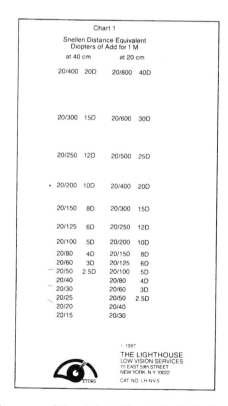

FIGURE 2-4 Close-up of the right side of the Lighthouse Near Visual Acuity Test Chart showing the predicted adds. (Courtesy Lighthouse Low Vision Products.)

that the Sloan method uses cards with continuous text sentences or paragraphs printed on them whereas the Lighthouse uses a card with lines of isolated letters.[2]

Example

A patient can read to the 4M line with a +2.50 add over the best-corrected prescription. Looking to the right side of the chart in the appropriate column (*at 40 cm*), you see that a +10.00 D add is indicated.

Discussion

With one assumption applied to the basic concept, we can derive the Lighthouse method. This assumption is that the desired acuity is 1M (20/50 Snellen equivalent at 16 inches). Note that the test is done at 16 inches with a +2.50 D add so the reference lens is +2.50. The formula for the basic concept thus becomes

$$\text{Predicted Add} = \frac{\text{M Value Read at Near}}{1} \times 2.50$$

which reduces to

$$\text{Predicted Add} = (\text{M Value Read})\,(+2.50)$$

Reciprocal of Vision

The Reciprocal of Vision method predicts an add based on both the patient's best-corrected distance acuity level and the actual desired near acuity level.

Method

A fraction is written with the present distance acuity level on top and the desired near acuity level on the bottom. This fraction is the same as the magnification ratio discussed previously (under the basic concept), and the conditions described there apply here. The fraction (ratio) is referred to as the *Reciprocal of Vision*. Multiply it by +2.50 D to get the predicted add for the patient's desired near acuity.[4] Note that this method suggests using a 20/40 goal for reading standard print, but any value can be put into the formula.

As originally taught, the top of the fraction is the denominator of the distance Snellen acuity and the bottom is the denominator of the reduced Snellen equivalent (referenced to 16 inches). Letter sizes in M notation can be substituted for the Snellen denominators.

Example

A patient reads 10/120 at far, measured with a Designs for Vision chart. The goal is to read footnotes in textbooks, and these are measured as 20/30 Snellen equivalent referenced to 16 inches. The Reciprocal of Vision is 240/30 = 8×. (Note that the numerator of the Reciprocal of

Vision is the denominator of the *20*-foot Snellen acuity [20/240]). Thus the predicted add is

$$8 \times 2.50 = +20.00 \text{ D}$$

In metric notation the distance acuity would be 48M at 4 meters (4/48) and the near desired acuity 0.6M at 40 cm (0.4/0.6). Translating the distance acuity to a near equivalent would give us 0.4/4.8 referenced to 40 cm. The Reciprocal of Vision fraction then becomes 4.8/0.6 = 8×, the same as found when using Snellen acuities.

Discussion

With two assumptions applied to the basic concept, we can derive the reciprocal of vision. These are that (1) distance and near acuities are equivalent and (2) the reference distance is 16 inches. The formula for the basic concept thus becomes

$$\text{Predicted Add} = \frac{\text{Distance Measured Snellen Denominator}}{\text{Near Desired Snellen Denominator}} \times 2.50$$

which is that given for the reciprocal of vision.

It should be noted that the reciprocal of vision allows a prediction of the add required for any task, not just reading. This can be done by substituting the acuity demand of the desired task into the formula to replace the reading acuity (in the denominator).

Analysis of 100 Clinical Records

You might ask: "How often do these methods predict the final add that is prescribed?" In an attempt to answer this question, 100 consecutive clinical records of low vision patients were examined and the following information was either recorded from the findings in the patient's record (marked with an r) or calculated from the findings based on the relationships given above (marked with a c):

1. Best-corrected distance acuity (r)
2. Lighthouse near test results (in M notation) (r)
3. Add predicted by Kestenbaum's rule (c)
4. Add predicted by Lighthouse method using the Lighthouse Near Visual Acuity Test chart (r)
5. Add predicted by reciprocal of vision (20/40 goal) (c)
6. Final add prescribed for the patient, or equivalent add if a hand-held or stand magnifier was prescribed (r)
   NOTE: The equivalent add is the single lens of comparable equivalent power that can replace the hand-held or stand magnifier when these are used with an add or accommodation.[5]

These data were recorded for the eye with the better visual acuity. The chart used for distance acuity was not specified, because the three methods do not require a specific distance chart. Based on this information, the following graphs were plotted:

1. Final add compared to the Kestenbaum predicted add (Fig. 2-5)
2. Final add compared to the Lighthouse predicted add (Fig. 2-6)
3. Final add compared to the reciprocal of vision predicted add (Fig. 2-7)

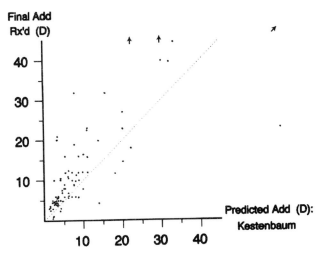

FIGURE 2-5 Results of a study using Kestenbaum's Rule to predict the add. *Arrows* indicate data points that fell outside the indicated range of the chart.

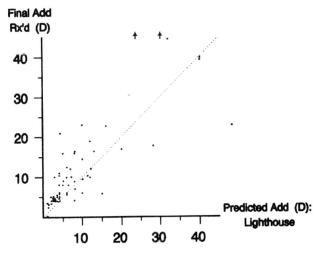

FIGURE 2-6 Results of a study using the Lighthouse Method to predict the add. *Arrows* indicate data points that fell outside the indicated range of the chart.

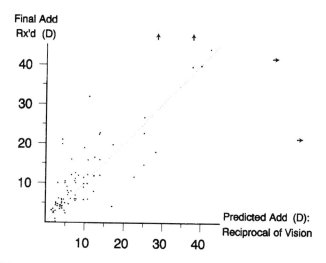

FIGURE 2-7 Results of a study using the Reciprocal of Vision method to predict the add. *Arrows* indicate data points that fell outside the indicated range of the chart.

Of the 100 records, 83 had information needed in the study. The others, for various reasons, could not be used. These reasons included that (1) the examination was not completed because the vision was too poor and (2) the patient did not return for completion of care, and the final prescriptions were thus not available. As a result the graphs for the Kestenbaum and reciprocal of vision methods have 83 plotted points. Only 62 records had the Lighthouse test results recorded, and the graph for this method therefore has only 62 entries.

Also shown on each graph is an "equality" line (i.e., where the predicted add and the final prescribed add are the same).

Results

Most of the final adds prescribed were of equal or greater value compared to the predicted add (Table 2-1).

In this analysis the reciprocal of vision method predicted the final add better than the other two did. This was most likely due to the use of a 20/40 goal, as opposed to the 20/50 goal assumed by the other two

TABLE 2-1

Method	Final add greater than predicted add (%)	Final add equal to or less than predicted add (%)
Kestenbaum	67 (81)	16 (19)
Lighthouse	45 (73)	17 (27)
Reciprocal of vision	52 (63)	31 (37)

methods, and it resulted in a higher predicted add and thus a closer correlation. In fact, if a 20/50 goal had been used in the calculation, the results would have been identical to those of the Kestenbaum method, since the Kestenbaum method also uses the distance acuity and assumes a 20/50 goal.

Although there can be many reasons why more of the final adds were greater than the predicted ones, the most likely are that (1) acuities were measured on high-contrast charts and (2) the acuities were taken with spread-out letters (not continuous text), thus reducing the effect of contour interaction. The final prescriptions were based on patient performance in tasks that usually included reading newspaper print (or at least not test charts). Newspapers are generally of lower contrast and the letters are printed close together. To get adequate performance in this type of task, it was not unusual to have to use a higher add. Some other considerations of varying importance included the patient's ability to move his or her eyes accurately across a line of print, the degree of eccentric viewing that might be present, the extent and location of visual field loss, the patient's binocularity, and the use of accommodation to augment the power of the add (resulting in holding the material closer than the add would have predicted or even holding the material closer, with a slight blur, to get the additional magnification). Also some patients might have significantly varied goals (e.g., reading large print books vs stock market quotations or baseball box scores).

Conclusions

It can be seen that the add predicted by these three methods will probably be on the low side. Whether this is a problem depends upon your evaluation style. If you want the patient to be able to read standard-sized continuous text print with the first lens tried, then either increase the value of the add predicted or use a smaller desired acuity as a goal (e.g., 20/30 instead of 20/40 in the reciprocal of vision method). One "clinical insight" based on our experience has been to increase the predicted add by about 30%. If you wish to start with a slightly weaker add than will finally be needed and work up to the full add, then starting with the predicted add will usually be appropriate.

CLINICAL PEARL

The add predicted by these three methods—Kestenbaum, Lighthouse, and reciprocal of vision—will probably be on the low side.

The main thing to remember is that the predicted add is a starting point. Patients vary significantly, and the final add prescribed will also vary significantly. The idea behind predicting an add is to get you started in your evaluation with a lens that should be close to the final lens prescribed.

References

1. Johnston A: Making sense of the M, N, and logMAR systems of specifying visual acuity. In Rosenthal B, Cole R (eds): *Problems in optometry: a structured approach to low vision care*, Philadelphia, 1991, JB Lippincott, vol 3, pp 394-407.
2. Fonda G: *Management of the patient with subnormal vision*, St Louis, 1965, Mosby, p 126.
3. Rosenthal B: The structured low vision evaluation. In Rosenthal B, Cole R (eds): *Problems in optometry: a structured approach to low vision care*, Philadelphia, 1991, JB Lippincott, vol 3, pp 389-390.
4. Newman JD (ed): *A guide to the care of low vision patients*, St Louis, 1974, American Optometric Association, pp 140-144.
5. Cole RG: A unified approach to the optics of low vision aids, I. *J Vis Rehabil* 2:23-36, 1988.

Appendix—A Look at Snellen Equivalent Acuities

Snellen visual acuity is still the most commonly used system of acuity notation in the United States today. There are certain situations, however, when the acuity fraction is misunderstood or even misused. Before looking at some specific situations, we should undertake a review of acuity notation.

Acuity Notation

Visual acuity is really a measurement of the resolution capability of the eye, or at least the ability of the eye to read the letters on the acuity chart, which we assume require a certain level of resolution capability. Our standard *20/20* assumes a minimum angle of resolution (MAR) of 1 minute of arc, *20/200* assumes an MAR of 10 minutes of arc, etc. In fact, the inverse of the Snellen acuity fraction gives the MAR. One way to specify acuity could be to write the MAR. The logMAR system of acuity notation uses the log of this MAR.

The key concept in recording visual acuity in any system other than MAR (or logMAR) is that you must record both the smallest letter size read and the distance at which it is read (test distance).

CLINICAL PEARL

The key concept in recording visual acuity is that you must record both the smallest letter size and the distance at which it is read (test distance).

The Snellen fraction gives both of these values:

$$\text{Snellen Acuity} = \frac{\text{Test Distance}}{\text{Letter Size Read}}$$

Test distance is the distance at which the letter is held. Letter size represents the distance at which this letter must be held to have an MAR of 1 minute (i.e., have the same visual angle as a "20/20" letter held at 20 feet). Note that letter size is a physical characteristic of the letter and does not vary with testing distance.

The units must be consistent. This means that if a test distance in feet is used, a letter size in feet must also be used. If the test distance is recorded in meters, the letter size must also be recorded in meters. For example, a 6M letter is one that subtends 5 minutes of arc at 6 meters. A person who can read only to a letter size of 6M when the chart is at 4 meters would have an acuity of 4/6. To translate this to Snellen acuity in feet (i.e., our standard "20 something" acuity), we have to multiply the top by a number to get 20 and then multiply the bottom by the same number. In this case we need to multiply the top by 5, so we also multiply the bottom by 5 and this gives us 30, or an acuity of 20/30. A person who gets 4/6 metric acuity has the same MAR as a person who gets 20/30 foot acuity. Although both are fractions, and can be thought of as Snellen fractions, it is customary to refer to acuities given in feet as Snellen acuities.

Some acuity charts give only the letter size (in feet or meters) and do not specify a test distance. These are the charts commonly used in low vision, in which the test distance can vary and is typically 10 feet, 4 meters, 2 meters, or even 1 meter. It is possible then to write the visual acuity as a fraction by writing the test distance used over the letter size read. Again, consistency of units in the fraction is essential.

Understanding the Lighthouse Distance Visual Acuity Test Chart

The Lighthouse Distance Visual Acuity Test Chart (Fig. 2-8) gives the letter size in meters for the far left column. The next column gives the

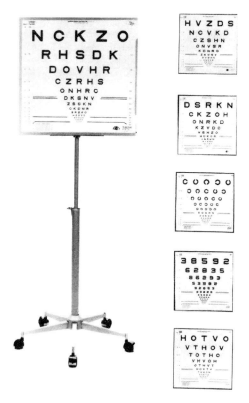

FIGURE 2-8 Lighthouse Distance Visual Acuity Test Chart. (Courtesy Lighthouse Low Vision Products.)

conversion to Snellen equivalent (Fig. 2-9). The purpose of this column is to allow you to quickly convert, without having to multiply, a metric acuity (e.g., 4/32) to a Snellen acuity that represents the same visual angle (MAR), in this case 20/160. As the instructions printed at the bottom of the chart indicate (Fig. 2-10), the number in this second column is to be used as the denominator of a Snellen acuity fraction, with a *20* in the numerator if the test is done at 4 meters, a *10* if the test is done at 2 meters, or a *5* if the test is done at 1 meter.

This is where a common error occurs. It is sometimes assumed that the second column is a letter size. **It is not.** The first column gives the actual letter size in metric notation: 40M for the top row. The correct letter size for this row in feet would be 131 feet (equivalent to 40 meters), **not** 200 feet. You cannot place this chart at 10 feet and record 10/200 for the top row, or place it at 5 feet and get 5/200 for the top row. The actual correct acuities would be 10/131 or 5/131, numbers a

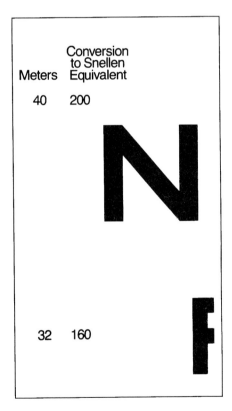

FIGURE 2-9 Close-up of the Lighthouse Distance Visual Acuity Test Chart showing the upper left corner. The first column is the letter size in metric notation, and the second column a conversion of the metric acuity to Snellen equivalent. (Courtesy Lighthouse Low Vision Products.)

Conversion to Snellen Equivalent

When testing at 4 meters, the numerator of the Snellen fraction is expressed as 20. Example: 20/200

When testing at 2 meters, the numerator of the Snellen fraction is expressed as 10. Example: 10/200

When testing at 1 meters, the numerator of the Snellen fraction is expressed as 5. Example: 5/200

FIGURE 2-10 Instructions printed on the bottom of the Lighthouse Distance Visual Acuity Test Chart giving the procedure for writing the Snellen equivalent of the metric acuity. (Courtesy Lighthouse Low Vision Products.)

little more difficult to work with. This chart is designed to be used with metric acuities, and it should be used this way.

One interesting point is that a 2-meter test distance allows the conversion to Snellen equivalent very easily. Just add a zero to the top and bottom numbers of the metric fraction: 2/32 metric thus becomes 20/320 in Snellen (feet). The 2-meter test distance also gives you an acuity range more appropriate for the low vision patient: 20/20 to 20/400 Snellen equivalent, instead of the 20/10 to 20/200 range when done at 4 meters. In addition, it is easier to point to the chart and work with the patient when the chart is 2 meters away instead of 4.

Understanding Near Acuities in Snellen Notation

Another common mistake in recording acuities happens with near acuities when Snellen notation is used. Near acuity charts having Snellen fractions printed on them are designed to be used at some specific test distance (e.g., often 16 inches [the standard test distance used by optometrists] but possibly other distances, such as 13 inches) (Fig. 2-11). One rotary card used with a phoropter has one set of Snellen acuities on it referenced to 16 inches and another referenced to 22 inches. Neither set is labeled with the reference distance.

Since near Snellen acuities are often written without the testing distance being indicated, you must assume that the standard test distance was used, **if you know this piece of information**. When 20/40 at near appears on a record, optometrists assume it means that the patient could read a letter subtending 10 minutes of arc (i.e., equivalent to the angular size of a [distant] 20/40 letter held at 20 feet). Thus we have the term *Snellen equivalent*. In fact, the Snellen fraction used at near can really be thought of as a letter size that correlates with the visual angle subtended by that letter when held at the standard test distance for which it was designed.

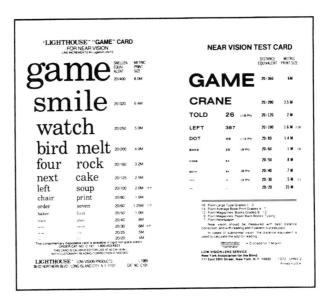

FIGURE 2-11 Two Lighthouse Near Vision Test Cards. The older one (*right*) is calibrated for 13 inches, and the newer one (*left*) for 16 inches. This can be seen by the Snellen equivalents (labeled *Distance Equivalent* on the older chart) written for the 1M lines: 20/60 (1M at 13 inches on the older card) and 20/50 (1M at 16 inches on the newer card). (Courtesy Lighthouse Low Vision Products.)

CLINICAL PEARL

The Snellen fraction used at near can really be thought of as a letter size.

If the near chart is held at any other distance, this should be specified (e.g., "20/40 at 8 inches" [actually "20/40 Snellen equivalent at 8 inches"]). This would mean that the patient can read the 20/40 equivalent line when the chart is held at an 8-inch distance. Realizing that the 20/40 equivalent line at 8 inches has the same visual angle as a 20/80 equivalent line at the 16 inch distance, we might say this patient has 20/80 acuity at near (or, more appropriately) 20/80 Snellen equivalent at near, assuming all acuities are referenced for a 16-inch distance.

If the test distance at near is not given, we must assume it. This is not the case in metric notation, in which acuities are recorded with distances (as 4M at 10 cm) or sometimes written as a Snellen-type fraction: 0.1/4. (Remember: Units have to be the same on both the top and the bottom of the acuity fraction—in this case, meters.)

3

Functional Vision Assessment of Infants

E. Eugenie Hartmann

Key Terms

Infant vision	Behavioral procedure	Visual evoked potential
Development	Preferential looking	Electrophysiology

Research on infant development has expanded tremendously in the last 30 years. In particular, studies of visual abilities in normal infants have been enhanced by the application and refinement of techniques designed to obtain quantitative answers regarding sensory processing from these nonverbal humans. Two major strategies have been implemented—behavioral and electrophysiological methods. The accumulation of data on normal visual development using these protocols has afforded application of this expertise to pediatric patient populations. The purpose of this chapter is to provide an overview of our current skills for evaluating visual abilities in human infants and young children with impaired visual processing.

Behavioral Testing

General Paradigm

Behavioral tests of visual acuity in pediatric patients (whether preverbal or nonverbal) are based on preferential looking (PL) techniques. Most of the early work using this technique was conducted by Fantz,[22-24] a developmental psychologist at Case Western Reserve University and his colleagues. Fantz's earliest work was intended to address the question of whether very young infants could discriminate between two different patterns. An independent observation of the phenomenon was also reported by Berlyne.[9]

In the PL technique, visual targets are presented to the infant in a display designed to minimize other distractions. Two stimuli are presented simultaneously. Generally the patterns are presented to the left and right of a central fixation point, spatially located in such a way that the infant's looking behavior will allow an observer to determine which pattern is being fixated. The reliability of the infant's "preference" for one pattern over the other is determined by the consistency or duration of looking, across a number of trials. This venue of research included comparisons between a variety of stimuli ranging from checkerboards and bulls-eyes to schematic human faces.[27] Early interpretations of these data led to speculations that infants' visual preferences were being driven by such dimensions as complexity of stimuli or number of contours.[26,34] The theoretical bases of these explanations were particularly unsatisfying and only later evaluated from a more rigorous perspective.[6,30] Nonetheless, using a behavioral technique, Fantz had achieved his goal of demonstrating rudimentary pattern perception in newborn infants.[25]

Applications to Acuity Testing

The first study of visual acuity using the PL technique was reported by Fantz, Ordy, and Udelf.[28] Their stimuli were black and white gratings paired with a gray target of equal space-average luminance. They used a total of five stripe widths ranging in size from 5 to 80 minutes of visual angle. Each pattern was presented twice, once to the infant's left and once to the right. The infant's responses were recorded as duration of looking time, number of fixations, and first fixation. Data from a group of infants were used to determine acuity estimates for infants aged 1 to 6 months. The results documented an improvement in visual acuity from approximately 20/800 in the 1-month-old group to 20/100 in the 6-month-old group.

The Forced-choice Preferential Looking (FPL) Procedure

A major limitation of the original PL technique was that estimates of visual acuity thresholds were not obtainable from individual subjects. The number of trials from a single subject was insufficient and therefore all results were reported as group data. A modification of Fantz's procedure was reported by Teller,[51] who combined the PL paradigm with a more conventional psychophysical procedure—the two-alternative forced-choice procedure (2AFC). This amalgamation became known as the Forced-choice Preferential Looking (FPL) procedure. The major advantage of this technique was the possibility of estimating an individual subject's visual threshold. For estimates of grating acuity using this procedure, an infant is shown black and white stripes paired with a gray stimulus of equal space-average luminance. The stimuli are presented to the right and to the left of a central peephole. An adult observer who cannot see the stimuli uses the infant's looking behavior to determine the location of the pattern on each trial. The observer's responses are objectively scored as correct or incorrect for each trial. A large number of stimuli are presented, usually five different stripe widths, each 20 times. This strategy is referred to as the method of constant stimuli. The data are plotted as observer's percent correct against stripe width. Acuity is estimated as the spatial frequency that yields a specified level of accuracy, conventionally set at a 75% correct criterion (Fig. 3-1).

The evolution of the FPL procedure allowed numerous researchers to explore the infant's visual sensory abilities. (Refer to several sources[2,5,52] for a general discussion of infant psychophysics.) This protocol also afforded the opportunity to evaluate an individual infant's

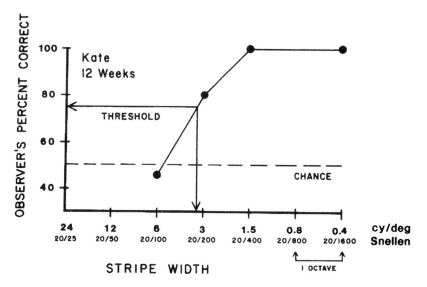

FIGURE 3-1 Psychometric function for an infant tested with the Forced-choice Preferential Looking procedure. Observer's percent correct is plotted for the four stripe widths used during the testing. Acuity threshold (*arrows*) is estimated as the stripe width (approximately 20/200) that produced 75% correct by the observer. Data points for the three smallest stripe widths are based on 20 trials per stripe width; for the largest stripe width the data point is based on 30 trials. (From Dobson V: *Int Ophthalmol Clin* 20:233-250, 1980.)

visual threshold, a prerequisite for use with any patient population. However, several aspects of the procedure made it unacceptable for widespread clinical application: The primary difficulty was its requisite number of trials. Even under ideal circumstances, at least 10 to 15 minutes were required to estimate one threshold. Typically, obtaining one threshold could be considered a full day's work for an individual infant. Monocular testing was mandatory for comprehensive clinical testing, requiring at least two threshold estimates. A technique for evaluating acuity that necessitated more than one session would obviously not be feasible in the majority of pediatric eye care practices. Other disadvantages with the procedure included the cumbersome nature of the stimuli and apparatus as well as the difficulty of obtaining complete data sets from infants older than 4 to 5 months. Although operant training techniques had been successfully integrated into the method for application with older infants,[38] the additions to the apparatus for this protocol were more rather than less complicated.

Modifications of the FPL Procedure

The earliest efforts to overcome the limitations of FPL testing for clinical applications tended to focus on strategies for decreasing the number of trials. One modification followed a staircase procedure, rather than the conventional method of constant stimuli.[32,36,39] With this procedure the stimulus presentation series depended on the subject's accuracy for each preceding trial.[12] Generally a two-down one-up staircase protocol was implemented. The starting point in the procedure was well above threshold. The strategy was to approach threshold over a series of trials and then concentrate a maximum number of trials around the threshold point.

Specifically, in this technique, after two correct responses the pattern is made more difficult (smaller stripes are presented) and after one incorrect response it is made easier. This results in a series of correct responses, moving to smaller and smaller patterns. Once threshold is approached, the responses tend to "staircase" around the threshold level. In a cooperative adult the technique can indeed lead to a need for fewer trials. For an infant, however, concentrating a maximum number of trials around the threshold point can actually be detrimental. These are the hardest stimuli for the infant to detect, and hence the most frustrating for both infant and observer. Although in theory the technique should yield a sensory threshold estimate in fewer trials, often the total number of trials to obtain a criterion number of staircase reversals is not noticeably different from that in the method of constant stimuli.

A second abbreviated protocol was the Diagnostic Stripe Width (DSW).[16,18-20] In this version of PL testing, a criterion pattern was established for a specific age group. The pattern was set as one that 90% of the normal population could detect. This approach allowed a rapid and qualitative assessment for an individual infant, but it did not provide a specific estimate of threshold.

The Acuity Card Procedure (ACP)

Finally, after extensive application of the FPL procedure in a number of laboratories, documenting the normative course of development of grating acuity in human infants, a major shift in testing approach unfolded. Teller and her colleagues developed the Acuity Card Procedure (ACP).[40-42, 53]

In the ACP, which incorporates a subjective judgment on the part of the observer, the stimuli and the presentation protocol are dramatically simplified. The earliest studies using this protocol have documented its validity and reliability. Data obtained using the subjective ACP are consistent with thresholds measured using the standard laboratory FPL (Fig. 3-2).

The acuity cards are gray with a black and white grating to one side of a central peephole. The cards are rectangular, measuring 25.5 by 55 cm. The grating measures 12.5 by 12.5 cm and is matched in space-average luminance to the background (i.e., the stripes cannot be discriminated from the background if the pattern is below an individual's acuity threshold). The width of the stripes varies from card to card. The largest pattern is 0.32 cycle/cm, and the smallest 38.0 cycles/cm. There are a

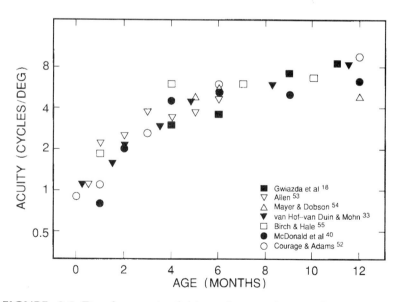

FIGURE 3-2 Development of binocular grating acuity in normal infants tested with three variants of the PL procedure—the method of constant stimuli,[3,32,38] a staircase procedure,[30,55] and the Acuity Card Procedure.[13,41] (From Dobson V. In Isenberg SJ: *The eye in infancy*, ed 2, St Louis, 1994, Mosby.)

total of 17 cards in a complete set,* including a low vision card and a blank card. The cards are presented to the subject through a window in a frame, which resembles a puppet stage (Fig. 3-3). This remodeling of the conventional laboratory stimuli has dramatically simplified the apparatus required for estimating visual acuity thresholds in infants.

The critical decrease in testing time with the ACP, however, resulted from a simple, though elegant, modification of the observer's task. In the FPL procedure the observer uses the infant's behavior to judge the position of the stimulus. The procedure generally limits the observer's response options to left or right. Although the accuracy of this objective response can be immediately evaluated, a great deal of information is being discounted by constraining the response in this manner. Highly experienced FPL observers quickly learn that an infant's looking behavior varies qualitatively with the difficulty of detecting the pattern, or how close the pattern is to the infant's threshold. For large patterns the infant tends to look quickly, directly, and for a relatively long interval

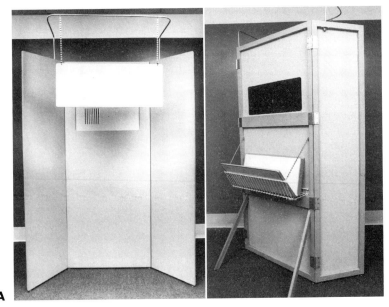

A   **B**

FIGURE 3-3 Apparatus for presenting Acuity Cards. **A**, Front view of the standing stage. Note the screen for occluding the holder's view of the stimulus pattern. **B**, Rear view of the stage showing the hanging basket for holding the cards during testing. (Children's Hospital and Medical Center, Seattle. Courtesy University of Washington, Department of Ophthalmology.)

*Available from Vistech Consultants, Dayton, Ohio, 45414.

in the direction of the pattern. If the observer were allowed to express a confidence rating for the accuracy of judgment in this case, it would undoubtedly be quite high. For small patterns, those close to threshold, the infant's looking behavior is much different. Under the FPL protocol an observer is often merely guessing the location of the pattern, with very low confidence in his or her judgment. In the ACP the observer is not only allowed but also required to utilize these qualitative components of the infant's looking behavior. Specifically, the observer's task is to evaluate whether an infant can detect the pattern. The observer's options are no longer "left" or "right" but rather "yes" or "no." This subtle alteration in response has provided a major breakthrough in the application of PL techniques for the evaluation of visual acuity in pediatric populations.

CLINICAL PEARL

Highly experienced Forced-choice Preferential Looking observers quickly learn that an infant's looking behavior varies qualitatively with the difficulty of detecting the pattern, or how close the pattern is to the infant's threshold. In the Acuity Card Procedure the observer is not only allowed but is required to utilize these qualitative components of the infant's looking behavior.

The ACP can be considered a "clinical method of adjustment." The observer starts with a pattern thought to be well above the individual's threshold. Although usually aware of the size of the pattern, the observer does not know its location. Based on the first presentation of a card, he or she can generate hypotheses about the pattern's location as well as whether or not the subject is able to detect the pattern. A second presentation with the card rotated 180° allows the observer to confirm his or her original speculation. If the fixation behaviors are rapid and alternate from side to side, the observer will infer that the pattern is above the individual's threshold, answering yes to the question "Can the child see the stripes?" This answer is validated by direct inspection of the card. If the observer is correct, the next card, with smaller stripes, is presented. Eventually a card will be presented that is below the subject's threshold. At this point the subject's behavior will be at best erratic. When a below-threshold card is presented to very young infants, they will often direct their gaze away from the screen, making it clear that there is nothing for them to look at. Threshold is specified as the last card to which the observer was willing to answer the ACP question with a definitive yes. Median duration required to obtain two monocular thresholds has been reported[37] as varying from 3.2 to 8.4 minutes across a wide age range (1 to 48 months) for normal subjects.

Modifications of the ACP for clinical testing

The advent of the ACP and concomitant development of the Teller Acuity Cards as a commercially available product have clearly impacted the quantitative assessment of visual functioning in pediatric populations. A comprehensive review of applications of the ACP with a variety of patient diagnostic categories is provided in a recent publication.[17] Strategies for maximizing success in the most difficult patient populations have evolved from the increasingly widespread use of the ACP. A number of subtle variations in technique for testing children with impaired vision have been presented.[54] (The first four authors of the treatise by Trueb et al.[54] were testers for a multicenter study and are particularly well qualified to present specific solutions. They obtained monocular grating acuities from hundreds of preterm infants for this study. Although some of these infants had normal vision, a number had partial or total retinal detachments due to retinopathy of prematurity [ROP] as well as a range of other ocular anomalies associated with prematurity.) These modifications of technique were all designed to obtain optimal performance from each infant.

Testing is often conducted away from the conventional stage for children with low vision. This allows the tester more flexibility in positioning the child as well as the cards and thus provides a more accurate assessment. Some infants will be more comfortable and cooperative when held over a parent's shoulder. Older children, especially those with other developmental problems, may be more comfortable in their own specially designed chairs. Evaluating the child's reaction to a direct view of the pattern versus a direct view of the gray field can be useful. The comparison—between presenting the child with a blank field and presenting the child with a pattern—often is sufficient in the hands of a skilled tester to evaluate the child's ability to detect the pattern. This protocol, referred to as *en face presentation*, is particularly helpful in children who have other motor impairments (e.g., cerebral palsy).[50] These children frequently display spontaneous random head/eye movements. Any subtle but consistent response to the stripes can be used to determine an acuity estimate.

CLINICAL PEARL

Testing is often conducted away from the conventional stage for children with low vision. This allows the tester more flexibility in positioning the child as well as the cards and thus provides a more accurate assessment.

The standard ACP involves horizontal presentation of the stimuli. Even when testing away from the puppet stage, an observer will hold the cards so the infant's gaze is directed either to the left or to the right to indicate detection of the pattern. Such horizontal shifts in fixation are quite difficult to observe in infants with spontaneous horizontal nystagmus. For these patients a vertical presentation of the cards will enhance the observer's ability to judge fixation behaviors. There is evidence[1,8] that adults with nystagmus have a higher threshold for horizontal stripes than vertical stripes. This difference may partly account for the observed improvement in visual acuity for nystagmus patients with vertical as opposed to horizontal presentations.[49] However, the ease of detecting upward and downward versus side to side fixations in these individuals cannot be underestimated. This variation may also be useful in patients with esotropia, who are often unable to abduct their esotropic eye when the stimulus is presented temporally. If an observer is looking for both a left and a right fixation, the shifts in direction of gaze may be too subtle. Again, vertical presentation will aid in successful completion of the testing.

CLINICAL PEARL

Horizontal shifts in fixation are quite difficult to observe in infants with spontaneous horizontal nystagmus. For these patients a vertical presentation of the cards will enhance the observer's ability to judge fixation behaviors.

The low vision card has been a valuable addition to testing materials. The pattern on this particular card consists of stripes that are 0.23 cycle/cm. Almost half the card is covered by the pattern. The appropriate scoring of acuity when using this card is not in cycles/degree (c/d) but rather at what specific distance the child is able to detect the card. The card is particularly useful for very young children with severely impaired vision and is virtually never presented in the stage (Fig. 3-4).

The manual for the Teller Acuity Cards lists specific start cards and test distances by age. These parameters apply to both normal subjects and some minimally affected infants. Testing a child with low vision, however, requires a certain sensitivity and awareness on the part of the observer. It is always advisable to start well above threshold when initiating a testing series. If the tester has started with a pattern that is clearly too easy for the child, cards can be skipped in the sequence to reach threshold more rapidly.

A variety of strategies are always employed for obtaining the child's attention. The tester usually has an array of noise-making toys as well as a number of repetitive vocalizations that he or she can employ to bring the child's direction of gaze to the center. For a patient whose vision is severely limited, pairing auditory and tactile stimulation with presentation of the visual stimulus can be extremely beneficial. One technique that may be exceptionally useful when working with a

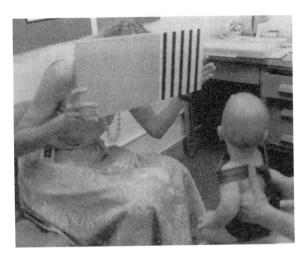

FIGURE 3-4 Assessment of pattern vision with the low vision card. The card, which contains a 25.5 × 23 cm area of 2.2 cm wide black and white stripes adjacent to a gray homogeneous field, can be presented in various parts of the visual field for an infant with severe visual acuity deficits. (From Dobson V. In Isenberg SJ: *The eye in infancy*, ed 2, St Louis, 1994, Mosby.)

child away from the puppet stage is to use the stimulus card as a fan. By rotating the card back and forth around the horizontal axis about 90°, the observer can generate a breeze. If this burst of air is immediately followed by presentation of the card (i.e., a visual stimulus), the child often learns to look for the pattern after feeling the breeze.

Summary

Establishment of the ACP represents the culmination of decades of research in laboratory settings. Application of the PL protocol with pediatric patients required an integrated effort and persistence between laboratory scientists and clinical practitioners. This example of the evolution of a technique from basic sciences to an applied clinical tool epitomizes the oft-stated goal of research endeavors. Furthermore, such achievements in the field of infant vision are manifestations of the quintessence of science. The establishment of a sound body of knowledge provides the basis from which clever and ingenious modifications of the PL technique are made not only valid but also profitable.

Electrophysiological Testing

Visual functioning in nonverbal individuals can also be evaluated using electrophysiological techniques, specifically the visual evoked potential (VEP). This test, a noninvasive measure of the visual system at the cortical level, entails recording brain wave activity that is synchronized with a visual stimulus. It is used to evaluate the integrity of the visual pathway from the retina to the visual cortex. Under appropriate conditions, it can be used to generate an acuity estimate. Stimuli can be either uniform flashes of light to generate a flash VEP (FVEP) or patterns to generate a pattern VEP (PVEP). For clinical purposes the FVEP may supply a measure of gross responsivity, which can be useful in limited circumstances.[47] However, FVEP responses often provide ambiguous or even contradictory information, and are therefore not useful in quantifying functional vision.[7,11,29] Extensive reviews of the VEP technique and its applications with infants for research as well as clinical purposes have recently been published.[33,44] The purpose of this discussion is to provide a general overview of the technique with particular emphasis on the application of PVEPs to a population of infants and young children with low vision.

CLINICAL PEARL

The visual evoked potential is considered a noninvasive measure of the visual system at the cortical level. It entails recording brain wave activity that is synchronized with a visual stimulus. It is used to evaluate the integrity of the visual pathway from the retina to the visual cortex. Under appropriate conditions, it can be used to generate an acuity estimate.

Types of Protocols

Conventional clinical testing protocols utilize counter phase reversing checkerboard patterns with a slow alternation rate. It is necessary to average a number of stimulus presentations to obtain a reliable response that is distinguishable from the underlying spontaneous EEG activity. At slow temporal frequencies (1 to 3 Hz) waveforms generated in response to these stimuli demonstrate characteristic peaks and troughs. The amplitude and latency of the positive-going peak that occurs approximately 100 msec after the stimulus onset is frequently used as a measure of visual response. This peak is commonly known as P100 (Fig. 3-5). The amplitude of the P100 peak has been shown to vary with stimulus size (Fig. 3-6). The absolute amplitude varies tremendously among individuals; however, the relative amplitude across checksizes or between eyes in a particular individual can provide meaningful information.

Recent advances in testing protocols have focused on techniques that yield rapid assessments of visual acuity and contrast sensitivity thresholds for application with infants.[44-46] The specific modification

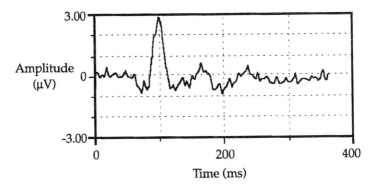

FIGURE 3-5 Transient VEP waveform elicited by a high-contrast checkerboard pattern. Data were obtained from a visually normal adult under the following stimulus conditions: binocular viewing, temporal frequency 2.7 Hz, checksize 80 minarcs, number of averages 163. Note the positive peak at 100 msec. Amplitude of the Nl-Pl peak, 3.5 µV. (From Hartmann EE: *Int J Neurosci* 80:203-235, 1995.)

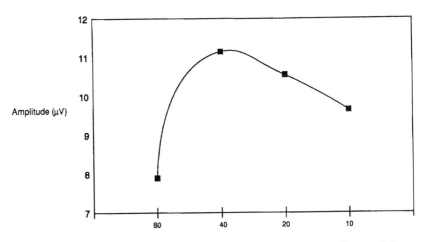

FIGURE 3-6 Plot of amplitude by checksize. Data were obtained from a visually normal adult under binocular viewing conditions. Patterns were phase-alternating checkerboards. Note the inverted U shape of the function. The amplitude is highest for a checksize of 40 minarcs and decreases with decreasing checksize. (From Hartmann EE: *Int J Neurosci* 80:203-235, 1995.)

developed by these researchers is known as the sweep VEP. Following this paradigm, stimuli are counterphase reversed at a moderate rate, usually 6 Hz. The size or contrast of the pattern is varied in rapid succession over a few seconds. Response waveforms are filtered on line using a discrete Fourier transform (DFT). The amplitude and phase of the second harmonic are analyzed across spatial frequency (or contrast), and a threshold estimate is derived by extrapolation to a specified criterion of noise. This analysis is provided in a software algorithm and can be conducted very rapidly (Fig. 3-7). Single sweeps can be repeated to evaluate consistency of the response, and vector averages are computed to utilize information from all trials.

The advantages of this sweep technique for rapid and accurate data collection with normal infants have been well documented.[44-46] Applications to clinical populations, however are scarce, particularly in contrast to the numbers of clinical studies that have used behavioral techniques.[17] One study[31] reported sweep VEP acuity estimates with 135 patients from a pediatric ophthalmology practice. The patients ranged in age from 3 weeks to 11 years (mean age, 4.3 years) and represented a wide variety of diagnostic categories, including amblyopia, strabismus without amblyopia, and retinal and optic nerve disorders. The authors concluded that the method provided estimates of acuity that corresponded well to other clinical findings. Results further documenting the utility of this testing in infants with infantile esotropia[14] and a multiply handicapped population[48] have been reported.

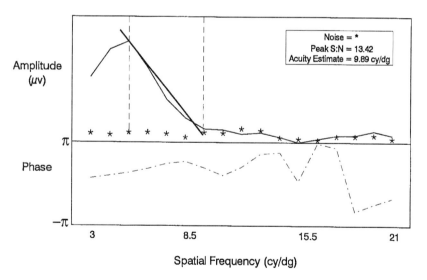

FIGURE 3-7 Plot of data from a single sweep VEP trial. Amplitude of the second harmonic (*2F*) plotted in microvolts against spatial frequency. Phase of component illustrated in the lower section of the graph. Data were obtained from a 20-week-old infant under the following stimulus conditions: binocular viewing, test distance 144 cm, spatial frequency sweep range 1 to 23 cycles/degree. The peak S:N ratio of 13.42 yields an acuity estimate of 9.89 c/d (Snellen equivalence 20/61), which is within normal limits for age. (From Hartmann EE: *Int J Neurosci* 80:203-235, 1995.)

Integration of Behavioral and Electrophysiology Tests

Several reports[4,35,48] have compared the use of both electrophysiological and behavioral techniques with populations of young children with low vision. The studies offered different conclusions concerning the relative success rates and utility of the two tests. The findings on multiply handicapped individuals ranging in age from 3 to 33 years reported by Orel-Bixler et al.[48] indicated a higher success rate with the sweep VEP technique than with behavioral testing (95% vs 70%). Their patients were much older than those tested in the other studies and the specific behavioral technique may not have been an optimal protocol. Bane and Birch[4] reported higher success rates with FPL testing than with VEP testing (98% vs 64%) in their population of 42 children ranging in age from 4 months to 9 years. In this instance the VEP testing was not conducted using a sweep protocol, which may have accounted partly for their poor success rate with that particular measure. However, the FPL technique was a staircase procedure that would have been expected to yield even poorer success rates than those reported. Finally, Katsumi et al.[35] measured visual function in 72 children between 6 and 49 months of age. They used a PL method that differed from the method used in the previously mentioned studies. Their VEP technique was similar to that implemented by Bane and Birch.[4] They concluded that the combination of testing protocols was more beneficial than relying on either protocol alone.

The reported inconsistencies in success rates when implementing both techniques provides a tantalizing challenge. None of these studies used optimal protocols for both procedures—ACP for behavioral testing and sweep VEP for electrophysiology testing. Clearly, there will be at least some individuals who are easier to test with one technique than the other. Based on the expense and training entailed in VEP testing, it remains more practical for most clinics to invest in behavioral testing as an initial strategy. With regard to the availability of data and the number of studies, comparisons between behavioral and electrophysiological techniques and their applications to clinical populations also remain biased in favor of behavioral testing. This discrepancy can be attributed to the equipment expense as well as the level of sophistication currently required for executing the two methodologies. Development of a VEP laboratory facility requires a major financial investment, well over a log unit more than that required for the commercially available behavioral testing apparatus (Teller Acuity Cards). Although mastery of the testing protocols for implementation of electrophysiological and behavioral testing may be equivalent, the technological skills required to sustain and develop the two laboratory facilities are quite disparate. Skilled technicians can obtain adequate results from a wide range of patients using the ACP. At the present time, the use of behavioral testing in clinical pediatrics is more widespread than the use of electrophysiology procedures. The technical expertise needed for successfully sustaining an electrophysiology laboratory remains illusive to the average, albeit skilled, technician. Masterful execution of a VEP protocol differs considerably from that required for responsible interpretation and presentation of the findings. Nonetheless, as advancing technologies lead to improved recordings and data analysis strategies as well as more innovative stimulus displays,[33,43] the VEP will manifest itself as a critical tool in the low vision clinic, especially with nonverbal populations.

Overview

In summarizing our understanding of visual abilities in young infants and the applications with a clinical population, certain limitations become apparent. A truly functional evaluation of a patient with low vision will ideally incorporate measures of the individual's abilities to adapt to his or her visual limitations and meet the demands of living in an able-sighted world. Interacting with a low vision patient, one is often struck by the extent to which the individual's behavior is visually driven. Infants and young children, in particular, who have never experienced a "normal" visual world demonstrate remarkable abilities to interact within the constraints of their experience. They have never seen objects or people in the detail we consider normal. Their entire development is based on the integration of a unique visual world with other senses. In evaluating the infant with low vision, perhaps it is the patient's ability to use visual input to function at an appropriate developmental level that should be considered. The visual function battery proposed in a recent study[21] is an example of a test that can rank severely visually impaired infants and young children whose acuities cannot be quantified even by the ACP but who clearly demonstrate visually driven interactions with their worlds. Further refinement of these innovative approaches remains the province of the researcher/clinician regularly involved in evaluations of this pediatric population.

CLINICAL PEARL

Infants and young children, in particular, who have never experienced a "normal" visual world demonstrate remarkable abilities to interact within the constraints of their experience. In evaluating the infant with low vision, perhaps it is the patient's overall development that should be considered more comprehensively.

References

1. Abadi RV, Sandikcioglu M: Visual resolution in congenital pendular nystagmus, *Am J Optom Physiol Opt* 52:573-581, 1975.
2. Abramov I: Whither infant psychophysics? In Simons K (ed): *Early visual development, normal and abnormal*, New York, 1993, Oxford University Press.
3. Allen JL: *The development of visual acuity in human infants during the early postnatal weeks.* Unpublished doctoral dissertation. Seattle, University of Washington, 1979.
4. Bane MC, Birch EE: VEP acuity, FPL acuity, and visual behavior of visually impaired children, *J Pediatr Ophthalmol Strabismus* 29:202-209, 1992.
5. Banks MS, Dannemiller JL: Infant visual psychophysics. In Salapatek P, Cohen L (eds): *Handbook of infant perception: from sensation to perception*, New York, 1987, Academic Press, Vol 1.
6. Banks MS, Salapatek P: Infant visual perception. In Haith M, Campos J (eds): Biology and infancy, pp. 435-571 in Musson P (ed): *Handbook of child psychology*, New York, 1983, Wiley.
7. Barnet AB, Manson JI, Wilner E: Acute cerebral blindness in childhood, *Neurology* 20:1147-1156, 1970.
8. Bedell HE, Loshin DS: Interrelations between measures of visual acuity and parameters of eye movement in congenital nystagmus, *Invest Ophthalmol Vis Sci* 32:416-421, 1991.
9. Berlyne DE: The influence of the albedo and complexity of stimuli on visual fixation in the human infant, *Br J Psychol* 49:315-318, 1958.
10. Birch EE, Hale LA: Criteria for monocular acuity deficit in infancy and early childhood, *Invest Ophthalmol Vis Sci* 29:636-643, 1988.
11. Bodis-Wollner I, Atkin A, Raab E, Wolkstein M: Visual association cortex and vision in man: pattern-evoked occipital potentials in a blind boy, *Science* 198:629-631, 1977.
12. Cornsweet TN: The staircase-method in psychophysics, *Am J Psychol* 75:485-491, 1962.
13. Courage ML, Adams RJ: Visual acuity assessment from birth to three years using the acuity card procedure: crossectional and longitudinal samples, *Optom Vis Sci* 67:713, 1990.
14. Day SH, Orel-Bixler DA, Norcia AM: Abnormal acuity development in infantile esotropia, *Invest Ophthalmol Vis Sci* 29:327-329, 1988.
15. Dobson V: Behavioral tests of visual acuity in infants, *Int Ophthalmol Clin* 20:233-250, 1980.
16. Dobson V: Clinical application of preferential looking measures of visual acuity, *Behav Brain Res* 10:25-38, 1983.
17. Dobson V: Visual acuity testing by preferential looking techniques. In Isenberg SJ (ed): *The eye in infancy*, ed 2, St Louis, 1994, Mosby.
18. Dobson V, Mayer DL, Lee CP: Visual acuity screening of preterm infants, *Invest Ophthalmol Vis Sci* 19:1498-1505, 1980.
19. Dobson V, Salem D, Mayer DL, et al.: Visual acuity screening of children 6 months to 3 years of age, *Invest Ophthalmol Vis Sci* 26:1057-1063, 1985.
20. Dobson V, Teller DY, Lee CP, Wade B: A behavioral method for efficient screening of visual acuity in young infants. I. Preliminary laboratory development, *Invest Ophthalmol Vis Sci* 17:1142-1150, 1978.
21. Droste P, Archer SM, Helveston EM: Measurement of low vision in children and infants, *Ophthalmology* 98:1513-1518, 1991.
22. Fantz RL: A method for studying early visual development, *Percept Mot Skills* 6:13-45, 1956.
23. Fantz RL: Pattern vision in young infants, *Psychol Rec* 8:43-47, 1958.
24. Fantz RL: The origin of form perception, *Sci Am* 204:66-72, 1961.
25. Fantz RL: Pattern vision in newborn infants, *Science* 140:296-297, 1963.

26. Fantz RL, Fagan JF: Visual attention to size and number of pattern details by term and preterm infants during the first six months, *Child Dev* 16:3-18, 1975.

27. Fantz RL, Fagan JF, Miranda SB: Early visual selectivity as a function of pattern variables, previous exposure, age from birth and conception, and expected cognitive deficits. In Cohen LB, Salapatek P (eds): *Infant perception: from sensation to cognition*, New York, 1975, Academic Press.

28. Fantz RL, Ordy JM, Udelf MS: Maturation of pattern vision in infants during the first six months, *J Comp Physiol Psychol* 55:907-917, 1962.

29. Frank Y, Torres F: Visual evoked potentials in the evaluation of cortical blindness in children, *Ann Neurol* 6:126-129, 1979.

30. Gayl IE, Roberts JO, Werner JS: Linear systems analysis of infant visual pattern preferences, *J Exp Child Psychol* 35:30-45, 1983.

31. Gottlob I, Fendick MG, Guo S, et al.: Visual acuity measurements by swept spatial frequency visual-evoked-cortical-potentials (VECPs): clinical application in children with various visual disorders, *J Pediatr Ophthalmology Strabismus* 27:40-47, 1990.

32. Gwiazda, J Brill, S Mohindra, I Held, R Infant visual acuity and its meridional variation. *Vision Res* 18:1557-1564, 1978.

33. Hartmann EE: Infant visual development: an overview of studies using visual evoked potential measures from Harter to the present. *Int J Neurosci* 80:203-235, 1995.

34. Karmel BZ: The effect of age, complexity, and amount of contour on pattern preferences in human infants, *J Exp Child Psychol* 7:339-354, 1969.

35. Katsumi O, Hirose T, Tsukada T: Evaluation and analysis of visual function in ROP (retinopathy of prematurity), *Am Orthopt J*, 39:112-124, 1989.

36. Lewis TL, Maurer D: Preferential looking as a measure of visual resolution in infants and toddlers: a comparison of psychophysical methods, *Child Dev* 57:1062-1075, 1986.

37. Mayer DL, Beiser AS, Warner AF, et al.: Monocular acuity norms for the Teller acuity cards between ages one month and four years, *Invest Ophthalmol Vis Sci.* 36:671-685, 1995.

38. Mayer DL, Dobson V: Visual acuity development in infants and young children as assessed by operant preferential looking, *Vision Res* 22:1141-1151, 1982.

39. Mayer DL, Fulton AB, Hansen RM: Preferential looking acuity obtained with a staircase procedure in pediatric patients, *Invest Ophthalmol Vis Sci* 23:538-543, 1982.

40. McDonald M, Dobson V, Sebris SL, et al.: The acuity card procedure: a rapid test of infant acuity, *Invest Ophthalmol Vis Sci* 26:1158-1162, 1985.

41. McDonald MA, Ankrum C, Preston K, et al.: Monocular and binocular acuity estimation in 18- to 36-month olds: acuity card results, *Am J Optom Physiol Opt* 63:181-186, 1986.

42. McDonald MA, Sebris SL, Mohn G, et al.: Monocular acuity in normal infants: the acuity card procedure, *Am J Optom Physiol Opt* 63:127-134, 1986.

43. Norcia AM: Improving infant evoked response measurement. In Simon K (ed): *Early visual development, normal and abnormal*, New York, 1993, Oxford University Press.

44. Norcia AM: Vision testing by visual evoked potential techniques. In Isenberg SJ (ed): *The eye in infancy*, ed 2, St Louis, 1994, Mosby.

45. Norcia AM, Tyler CW: Infant VEP acuity measurements: analysis of individual differences and measurement error, *Electroencephalogr Clin Neurophysiol* 61:359-369, 1985.

46. Norcia AM, Tyler CW, Hamer RD: Development of contrast sensitivity in the human infant, *Vision Res* 30:1475-1486, 1990.

47. Odom JV, Chao G, Hobson R, Weinstein GW: Prediction of post cataract extraction visual acuity: 10 Hz visually evoked potentials, *Ophthalmic Surg* 19:212-218, 1988.

48. Orel-Bixler DA, Hagerstrom-Portnoy G, Hall A: Visual assessment of the multiply-handicapped patient, *Optom Vis Sci* 66:530-536, 1988.

49. Raye K, Pratt E, Rodier D, et al.: Acuity card and grating orientation: acuity of normals and patients with nystagmus, *Invest Ophthalmol Vis Sci (Suppl)* 32:960, 1991.

50. Rodier D, Raye K, Mayer DL: Unconventional acuity card testing: tester reliability and notable cases, *Invest Ophthalmol Vis Sci (Suppl)* 34:1422, 1993.

51. Teller DY: The forced-choice preferential looking procedure: a psychophysical technique for use with human infants, *Infant Behav Dev* 2:135-153, 1979.

52. Teller DY: Psychophysics of infant vision: definitions and limitations. In Gottlieb G, Krasnegor NA (eds): *Measurement of audition and vision in the first year of postnatal life: a methodological overview*, Norwood NJ, 1985, Ablex.

53. Teller DY, McDonald MA, Preston K, et al.: Assessment of visual acuity in infants and children: the acuity card procedure, *Dev Med Child Neurol* 28:779-789, 1986.

54. Trueb L, Evans J, Hammel A, et al.: Assessing visual acuity of visually impaired children using the Teller acuity card procedure, *Am Orthopt J* 42:149-154, 1992.

55. Van Hof-van Duin J, Mohn G: The development of visual acuity in normal fullterm and preterm infants, *Vision Res* 26:909-916, 1986.

4

Pathology and Visual Function

Eleanor E. Faye

Key Terms

Vision rehabilitation	Brightness acuity	Macular
Low vision history	testing	degeneration
Amsler grid	Binocular testing	Advanced glaucoma
Contrast sensitivity	Function tests	Retinitis pigmentosa
function	Cataract	Diabetic retinopathy

Successful low vision practice requires a commitment to the concept of visual rehabilitation. A careful history should be taken emphasizing the patient's coping skills and visual objectives. Function tests should include Amsler grid, contrast sensitivity, and glare. Remember: eye pathology affects the patient's response to low vision devices; for example, macular degeneration leaves the periphery free to receive a magnified image whereas glaucoma reduces both the peripheral receptors and macular function, which in turn reduces the response to magnification. A prescription should take into consideration the patient's response to function tests as well as the eye pathology and the realistic task objectives that the patient has before him.

A vision rehabilitation program is geared toward uncovering the effect of eye disease on visual function, the level of motivation, and the specific visual requirements of the patient for daily activities. The devices and products that are needed to achieve better visual performance are recommended after an evaluation of several areas of visual function.

The patient receives instruction in the use of visual aids until a satisfactory skill level is reached, and then a prescription is made.

Another consideration is general health—the presence of medical conditions that could delay or diminish the rehabilitation process and increase the need for counseling or other social intervention.

One of the first problems to be tackled is the degree of knowledge or insight a patient has concerning the eye condition, its course, and its prognosis. Many ophthalmologists, while dealing competently with diagnosis and treatment in the acute phase, are not aware of the patient's reaction to diminished sight. The low vision evaluation process cannot be effective until misunderstandings, unrealistic hopes, and very real fears are dealt with in the early stages of the history.

An understandably depressed person should be allowed to ask questions about the eye disease, about its treatment, and about the feelings of frustration that are inherent in the experience of losing sight.

The doctor should realize that a patient is not putting him or her "on the spot," does not really expect miracles, but wants to be allowed to seek reassurance and to be told what to expect realistically from the disease and the rehabilitation plan. Patients do not need a dissertation as much as they need action.

The History

The history establishes a doctor/patient relationship that facilitates the therapeutic effect. For the low vision patient a brief review of the history is an excellent time to pinpoint areas of personal difficulty and the impact of the disease on the person's life. During history taking, encourage the patient to discuss reactions and fears directly. Usually the realization that problems can be aired and talked about, even briefly, starts the therapeutic ball rolling.

Some subjects of interest to the patient might be the role of nutrition and vitamin supplements, the effect of medications, and the possible underlying cause of the disease. If the disease had an acute onset, you might try to identify an event that precipitated it. What chronic stress could have made the patient susceptible? Patients often feel that they are "to be blamed" and may even identify a particular event as the cause. You should listen for clues in the medical history that suggest answers that would be most reassuring.

If you are doing the evaluation, you should also be the one who takes the history. A medical history is actually a recital of personal data, reactions, and feelings known only to the patient. You need to listen with a "third ear," storing sensitive data for future use and pursuing significant answers with further questions if the patient's answers affect the treatment plan.

You also can use phrases such as "How did you feel about that?" or "What was your reaction?" or "How have you coped with the problem?" This need not be time consuming if you understand that you can still control the flow of the examination by guiding the patient to answer appropriately. A history that explores all avenues of the patient's concerns makes the remainder of the evaluation more meaningful to the patient.

> **CLINICAL PEARL**
>
> *A history that explores all avenues of the patient's concerns makes the remainder of the evaluation more meaningful to the patient.*

Tests

Of increasing importance to the low vision clinician are tests of visual function used to augment conventional visual acuity and reading tests. Function tests may identify potential problems with the use of magnifying devices.

Binocular Testing

Keep in mind this basic principle: Most low vision patients, if born with normal oculomotor function, continue to use both eyes in tandem. Field deficits do not necessarily disrupt the use of binocular cues, and patients often report the "filling in" effect of one eye helping the other. Nevertheless, tests are most often administered *monocularly*, and seldom are binocular results noted.

Tests that can be performed binocularly (visual acuity, Amsler grid, contrast sensitivity) are valuable indicators of the effect of pathology on the patient's binocular response and the influence of the dominant eye when both eyes are used together. Recent improvements in test procedures, and the accumulation of data from tests developed during the 1980s, have proved the importance of including these tests in a comprehensive low vision evaluation. Function tests should be administered after the refraction and near vision evaluation but before any low vision aids are introduced.

> **CLINICAL PEARL**
>
> *Tests that can be performed binocularly (visual acuity, Amsler grid, contrast sensitivity) are valuable indicators of the effect of pathology on the patient's binocular response and of the influence of the dominant eye when the eyes are used together.*

The monocular glare test is introduced if cataracts or corneal pathology complicates the picture.

Visual Acuity

Starting with vision tests and refraction, you can often improve sight (somewhat or significantly) by a review of refraction and a binocular assessment. By testing the acuity in both eyes separately, and then together, comparing the old refraction with the new in a real-life setting, you will be able to make a fairer assessment of any improvement that is achieved.

Binocular improvement is significant in itself, but it may also suggest an eventual trial of binocular reading lenses (e.g., base-in prism half-eye glasses) or a closed-circuit television (which is viewed with both eyes). A *reduction* in acuity on binocular testing may suggest the need for occlusion of the dominant poorer eye and a monocular optical aid.

Reading Acuity

Reading is a significant visual function test, and reading skills should be assessed early in the evaluation using graded prose text selections, such as Lighthouse or Bailey cards.[1] Not only will reading skill be tested, but binocular potential can also be evaluated.

Case example

Mr. H. H., a 63-year-old writer, came in complaining that he was having difficulty reading with the +18 aspheric lens that had been prescribed for his left eye. Near acuity OD was 5M (20/250), and OS was 4M (20/200). Binocularly with graded text he read 2M (20/100). He accepted binocular half-eye prism glasses, +8 with 10 base-in prism, which enabled him to easily read 0.8M (20/40) print.

Visual Fields

Automated visual fields are not customarily tested binocularly, but you can superimpose the two monocular field charts to see how corresponding areas overlap and "fill in" for a scotomatous area. Another example of a helpful test is the threshold automated macular field that expresses responses digitally and can demonstrate the variability in depth of macular pathology. You may be able to identify the proportion of better areas in each field and thus predict the macular response better. With the advent of scanning laser ophthalmoscopy it has become possible to identify areas of best function more directly.

Amsler Grid

The Amsler grid, though not intended originally as a clinical tool for low vision evaluations, serves several useful purposes:
  1. Locating a scotoma. If a patient with a macular lesion continues to fixate foveally, the central fixation target of the grid will be obliterated or faded. But if the patient has adapted to eccentric viewing, the fixation dot will be clearly seen. This is a good prognostic sign, unless the major distortion or loss of grid boxes is just

to the *right* of fixation (which interferes with scanning). Scotomas above, below, and to the left of fixation have a better prognosis for response to magnification.

2. Sizing a scotoma. If the patient has a large scotoma centrally, response to magnification will be questionable unless the scotoma can be shifted away from fixation.

3. Demonstrating the dominant eye. A patient's dominant eye may also be demonstrated on the Amsler grid (Fig. 4-1). The two similar grid patterns in this figure demonstrate why binocular testing is critical. In the second example (in which the left eye is dominant) binocular correction would be appropriate. In the first example, occlusion of the right eye would be more appropriate.

 CLINICAL PEARL

The Amsler grid, although not intended originally as a clinical tool for low vision evaluations, serves several useful purposes—locating a scotoma, sizing a scotoma, and demonstrating the dominant eye.

Method

With best correction and a +3.00 add OU, present the grid at 33 cm binocularly. Ask, "Can you see the dot?" If the answer is yes, it indicates either a small functional central area or that the patient has learned to use another retinal locus. To gain further information, ask

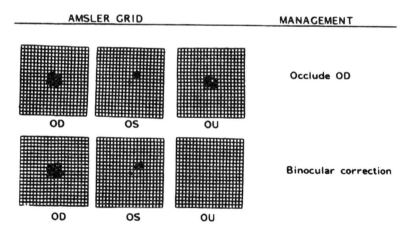

FIGURE 4-1 In the first example the right eye, with the larger scotoma, is dominant. The test OU suggests a need for occlusion OD. In the second example the left eye is dominant and the test OU is negative, which suggests trial of binocular rather than monocular reading glasses.

the patient to look *directly* at the dot. If that maneuver blots out the fixation point, you can assume that the patient has been using a parafoveal area binocularly. Next, check each eye separately and then return to and compare the binocular response. By seeing the pattern of their macular pathology, patients are often better able to monitor changes in the grid pattern over time if they use an Amsler grid at home.

Results on a grid can corroborate findings from automated fields and explain difficulties in reading. Having several sources of data leads you toward a prescription that is appropriate for the pathology or explains (or predicts) failure or poor performance. You will be prevented from making too-optimistic statements early in the evaluation and be forewarned of difficulties.

Contrast Sensitivity Function

Since the introduction of a practical clinical test for contrast sensitivity function (CSF) by Ginsberg[2] and the subsequent development of new tests,[3,4] there has been increased understanding of the importance of the CSF in low vision evaluation.

The concept of a retina that is not simply geared to one high frequency (i.e., visual acuity) but functions at many frequencies and intensities of stimuli, even outside the fovea, has changed our concept of eye disease. We now look at each disorder to determine what frequencies and contrast levels have been affected. The binocular response provides valuable information about the level of contrast the patient may require for reading or getting about in the environment. Test the better eye first. After the fellow eye has been tested, binocular evaluation (as with the acuity and grid) is needed to tell you more about the patient's visual concept of the real world and to help anticipate problems reading with the optical device you have prescribed as well as identifying objects in the surroundings.

CLINICAL PEARL

The concept of a retina that is not simply geared to one high frequency (i.e., visual acuity) but functions at many frequencies and intensities of stimuli, even outside the fovea, has changed our concept of eye disease.

Method

With best correction (and a +1.00 add if it improves acuity) present the Vistech 6500 at 1 meter. Show the patient the test circles binocularly, describing the patches as tilted left, tilted right, vertical, or blank and requesting verbal or hand position responses. Proceed monocularly with the better eye (previously determined by acuity and the Amsler grid) and then the fellow eye. To complete the test, compare these findings with the binocular response, starting at the level of the best monocular answer (Fig. 4-2). The binocular response is more significant than the response of either eye alone, usually being better than the monocular test because of the summation effect; if it is worse, however, the poorer eye should be occluded when reading or for distance, if it interferes.

Case example

The macular degeneration patient in Figure 4-2 was unhappy reading with a monocular lens of +20 that had been prescribed. Monocular contrast OD and OS showed subnormal curves, with only three targets seen by OS. Binocularly,

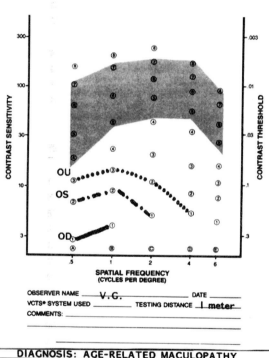

OBSERVER NAME ____V.G.____ DATE _____

VCTS® SYSTEM USED _____ TESTING DISTANCE __1 meter__

COMMENTS: _____

DIAGNOSIS: AGE-RELATED MACULOPATHY

VA: OD 8/200   OS 10/200

OU 10/100

CSF: OD 1-1-0-0-0

OS 2-2-1-0-0

OU 3-3-2-1-0

RX: +12 w 14 prism diopters base-in OU

Had been wearing +20 OS

FIGURE 4-2 Contrast sensitivity testing at 1 meter shows binocular reinforcement of the contrast curve. A +20 monocular reading lens had been prescribed OS on the basis of a monocular visual acuity of 10/200. Binocularly the patient accepted a reading add of only +12.00 D with 14 Δ base-in OU.

however, the contrast increased to a level at which a binocular correction for reading was feasible. The patient responded to a binocular half-eye prism of +12 with 14 Δ base in OV.

Glare Test

A practical and simple glare test to administer is the Brightness Acuity Test (BAT) (made by Mentor). If a patient has a cataract complicating retinal or optic nerve pathology, this test may be helpful in suggesting the ultimate response to surgery. In Table 4-1, though, a negative BAT test is illustrated. Be sure to confirm that the patient does not have any complaints. In Table 4-2 a positive effect of glare is documented. This patient had not remembered to comment on glare sensitivity until the test was administered, and his response to the test was, "This is just what it's like outside on a sunny day!"

Importance of Function Tests

Because tests must be relied on to help plan treatment, they should be used appropriately, with the patient's understanding and cooperation. They will help you determine the type and strength of device to use

CLINICAL PEARL

Function tests help you determine the type and strength of device to use and also present the disease process in functional terms that a patient can actually see.

TABLE 4-1
Negative Brightness Acuity Test (BAT)

	Baseline	Low	Medium	High
	OD 20/50	20/60	20/80	20/80
	OS 20/40	20/50	20/60	20/70

The diagnosis here was nuclear cataract. In this essentially negative test the acuity reduction is two lines on a Snellen chart.

TABLE 4-2
Positive Brightness Acuity Test

	Baseline	Low	Medium	High
	OD 20/50-2	20/60	20/80	20/300
	OS 20/40	20/50	20/100	20/400

The diagnosis here was anterior cortical cataract. With this defect, light is refracted in a random fashion and also present the disease process in functional terms that the patient can actually see. Patients who see their scotoma on a grid or know that the contrast test has confirmed their problem with stairs and curbs will be more knowledgable participants in the treatment plan.

Management of Specific Eye Conditions

Cataract

For low vision patients, cataract is a secondary and unwelcome complication because it adds other symptoms (blur, haze, photophobia) to those of the primary disease.

The surgeon is faced with a dilemma: Are the patient's visual complaints due to macular degeneration, glaucoma, diabetic retinopathy? Or are they the result of the cataract? Evaluation consists of observing the cataract for its position (nuclear, subcapsular) and density, reviewing the visual fields, intraocular pressure, and fluorescein angiogram, and then conducting glare tests. Informal assessment of glare with a flashlight or bright window light is less reproducible than a test such as the Mentor BAT. A rapid decline in Snellen acuity with the BAT is reliable, since only interference of the lens or a corneal opacity gives the responses illustrated in Tables 4-1 and 4-2.

Patients generally can respond to a glare test because it relates to their own experience. While they are in the subdued light of your office, they may say that their vision indoors is no problem, but they fail to mention what happens outdoors.

Anterior cortical cataracts with spokes crisscrossing the pupil usually respond dramatically to glare testing (Table 4-2). A posterior subcapsular cataract will respond according to its size and whether it is fibrous or vacuolated. Vacuolated opacities often act as tiny prisms, creating a glare. Nuclear cataract patients may have a relatively normal glare test (Table 4-1).

Before recommending surgery, be sure that alternative treatments have been attempted. For example, in a patient with a cortical cataract, try light to medium gray wraparound sunglasses, visors, or a cap. For the patient with a nuclear cataract, dilating the pupil or providing a light gray lens to reduce light intensity may prove efficacious.

When cataract surgery has been recommended, implants are indicated. However, risk factors must be seriously considered and discussed with the patient—e.g., a poor result in the fellow eye, fear of surgery, the need for anticoagulant drugs, the possibility of pulmonary obstructive disease, and the potential for retinal bleeding in "wet" macular disease and diabetic retinopathy. Patients should be in optimal health, on a sound nutrition program, and aware of the fact that only the cataract symptoms will be alleviated not their basic eye problem.

Macular Degeneration

The prevalence of macular degeneration in all statistics is a major source of concern among clinicians involved with low vision clinical care. Although diagnostic tests and laser treatment have made remarkable progress in recent decades, the fact remains that most patients do not maintain their acuity level and most are over 65. Patients often must deal with a substantial adjustment in their lives at a time when they are ill equipped to do so.

You need to spend additional time with older patients, reviewing the areas of strength in their lives that might provide a positive atmosphere and the assistance they need to keep up their energy and to move into a new way of using sight. The general health evaluation should deal specifically with cholesterol and lipid levels, ruling out anemia, the side effects of medications, and the possibility of noncompliance with therapeutic regimens. Sensible nutritional advice can give a patient some feeling of being in control. Many patients request advice about antioxidant vitamins and other nutritional agents that appears in current periodicals.

Macular degeneration patients usually are told that they will not be blind. But they need additional positive reinforcement. A low vision evaluation should be offered, and the value of residual vision should be emphasized rather than dwelling on what has been lost. What is left can and should be used. One depressed patient was helped by her ophthalmologist, who said to her, "You have two choices: you can sit at home and rot, or you can get out and live." She chose the latter, embarking on a program of weight reduction and exercise, and began to participate more in family and other social activities.

Hope should not be false, however. It is false if it is meant only to pacify the ill person. True hope stems from a patient's discovery that life can be controlled in some fashion. With attention to health and exercise, and the use of magnifying or other visual or audio aids, an individual can work gradually toward a new meaning in life and can reach an equilibrium with this disease.

CLINICAL PEARL

With attention to health and exercise, and to the use of magnifying or other visual aids, patients with macular degeneration can work gradually toward a new meaning in their lives and can reach an equilibrium with their disease.

The patient may wish to visit a counselor or have a low vision evaluation at an agency for the blind and visually impaired. Most agencies for the "blind" now deal with a majority of sighted clients. Unfortunately, over the years when blindness was more prevalent, agencies tended to develop a specific technology for blind people and came only slowly to realize that their mission was to assist the seeing-impaired as well. You should not hesitate, however, to refer this person to such an institution because of the possibility that you might be delivering a message that you really believe blindness is the ultimate fate and are trying to let the patient down gently.

If the best low vision counseling and rehabilitation services are available from an agency for the "blind," you should be forthright in telling the patient that there is no hidden agenda: this is an agency that will provide services to support your work, services that you cannot offer.

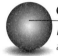

CLINICAL PEARL

If the best low vision counseling and rehabilitation services are available from an agency for the "blind," you should be forthright in telling the patient that there is no hidden agenda: this is an agency that will provide services to support your work, services that you cannot offer.

Support groups may help, as may talking things over with another person (frequently a sibling or a friend who has the same condition).

Patients who remain depressed and negative after the prescription of a low vision device may need counseling in other areas of their lives, as well as an evaluation for antidepressant medication.

Advanced Glaucoma

Among the most difficult diseases to evaluate and treat is advanced glaucoma with massive nerve fiber layer damage. Not only is acuity affected, but contrast sensitivity is reduced and large areas of visual field may be obliterated so that conventional magnifying aids are often not effective. In such cases, when the CSF is obviously well below normal threshold, improving contrast with yellow lenses (Corning 450, 511; NoIR yellow or light amber), yellow acetate paper over print, or high-level nonglare illumination may help. Closed-circuit television magnifying reading machines with white print on a dark background may in some cases provide the best contrast.

CLINICAL PEARL

Advanced glaucoma is difficult to evaluate and treat, since not only is acuity affected but contrast sensitivity is reduced and large areas of visual field may be obliterated so that conventional magnifying aids often are not effective.

Many glaucoma patients require mobility instruction and can benefit from talking aids (e.g., clocks, computers, tapes, reading machines).[5]

Retinitis Pigmentosa

The problems that arise for a patient with advanced retinitis pigmentosa (RP) are related to the size of the central field and the presence of cataract. Cataract is an underrated complication in RP patients who have residual fields so small that their mobility is limited. The posterior subcapsular cataract commonly starts in the patient's 30s, yet it may not be removed until it reaches the 2 to 3 mm size. If a glare test is done at the first sign of an opacity and is followed at yearly intervals (or more often), it soon becomes apparent that a 1.5 mm central posterior subcapsular cataract effectively blocks vision in a field occupying less than 10°. Cataract extraction should be performed as soon as visual function is restricted, and an IOL should be implanted. It frequently is good judgment in an RP patient to insert an implant that overcorrects by about 3 D. The resulting myopia will be useful in the near reading range and can easily be corrected for distance.

CLINICAL PEARL

A posterior subcapsular cataract is an underrated complication for retinitis pigmentosa patients who have residual fields so small that their mobility is limited. A relatively small opacity can cause blurred vision throughout the field.

If the central field is less than 6°, response to magnification will be limited. And if the central acuity is reduced because of additional macular pathology, mobility is likely to be compromised.

Reading fields are easily measured on an Amsler grid at the patient's reading distance, using a small white test object and taking care to prescribe the least amount of magnification for the size of the field.

Diabetic Retinopathy

The factors that make diabetes a problem in management are the effects of extensive laser treatment, the progressive nature of the disease, and the need for cooperation among ophthalmologist, diabetologist, retinologist, and low vision specialist. Probably more than any other patients, diabetics experience loss of control over their lives and medical condition. Despite the fact that it tends to reduce night vision and contrast, laser photocoagulation of the retina has been shown to delay the development of proliferative retinopathy. Medical problems include peripheral circulatory and cardiovascular disease, overweight, hyperglycemia, and hypercholesterolemia. If blood sugar is difficult to control, patients may need frequent hospitalizations. They also may have to face vitreous surgery, with prolonged visual recovery, and surgery for detached retina.

One mission of the low vision specialist is to follow the diabetic patient closely in conjunction with other specialists, so the patient never experiences prolonged visual dysfunction after vitreous or retinal surgery. Magnifying aids and good lighting can be supplied and changed whenever required.

CLINICAL PEARL

One mission of the low vision specialist is to follow the diabetic patient closely in conjunction with other specialists, so the patient never experiences prolonged visual dysfunction after vitreous or retinal surgery. Magnifying aids and good lighting can be supplied and changed whenever required.

Patients should be encouraged to seek consultation with an ophthalmologist who specializes in diabetic vitroretinal conditions and to take control of their lives by understanding their disease, its hazards, and its consequences.

Conclusion

Problems in the patient with low vision may be related directly to the physical characteristics of the disease or indirectly to the adjustment factors. If you wish to avoid the frustrating aspects of caring for patients with low vision, you would do well to perform function tests to analyze the disease process in each individual and help your patients understand both the disease process and how to direct their inner strengths toward living with a disease that will never go away.

Low vision evaluation—visual rehabilitation, including life adjustment and low vision devices—is the optical component of medical/surgical eye care. And as such, it becomes the responsibility of both optometry and ophthalmology.

References

1. The Lighthouse Inc: *Lighthouse low vision catalog*, ed 9, New York, 1994, The Lighthouse.
2. Ginsburg AP: A new contrast sensitivity chart, *Am J Optom Physiol Opt* 61:403-407, 1984.
3. Evans DW: Contrast testing now easy, *Contrast Sensitiv Update*, Spring 1990, Vol 3.
4. Hyvarinen L: Contrast Sensitivity Function Test, 1979.
5. The Lighthouse Inc: *Consumer products catalog 1994-95*, New York, 1994, The Lighthouse.

5

Next Generation Contrast Sensitivity Testing

Arthur P. Ginsburg

Key Terms

Visual acuity	Low-contrast letter	VCTS
Contrast	charts	SWCT
Contrast sensitivity	Sine-wave grating	FACT
Visual channels	contrast sensitivity	Functional vision
Low-contrast letter	charts	EyeView
acuity		

Contrast sensitivity testing is gaining increased recognition as a valuable tool for measuring functional vision. It can successfully detect functional vision loss, often caused by early eye disease, and has been proven[1-5] to provide a more sensitive and comprehensive measurement of visual capability and performance than is provided by Snellen visual acuity.

There are several contrast test systems available. Each has a specific format, application, delivery system, and scoring procedure—therefore generating different information about the visual system.

One key difference in the test technologies is the target type. Sine-wave grating measures specific visual channels, providing a contrast sensitivity curve that is more comprehensive and informational than the less specific results obtained from low-contrast letter acuity systems.

We will review some advantages and disadvantages of each approach to contrast testing and demonstrate how the various tests can be compared to understand important differences between them. We will also discuss some contrast test display issues and illustrate how visual acuity and contrast sensitivity data can be used to create pictures of how some people "see."

Sine-Wave Grating and Low-Contrast Letter Charts

Although sine-wave gratings have been the most widely used test targets in visual psychophysics for the last 29 years, it was the introduction of sine-wave grating charts that launched contrast sensitivity out of the laboratory into the clinical and applied research environment. The Arden grating[6] quickly gave way to the Vision Contrast Test System (VCTS, Vistech Consultants)[7] as a simple, quick, and inexpensive way to create and measure a contrast sensitivity curve. Recently, the next generation of VCTS-type charts has become available using computer-generated sine-wave gratings for improved quality—the Sine-Wave Contrast Test (SWCT, made by Stereo Optical), similar to the VCTS, and the Functional Acuity Contrast Test (FACT, Stereo Optical).

The FACT (Fig. 5-1) was developed to improve the sensitivity and quality of the VCTS. The possibility of aliasing from the VCTS—spurious phantom gratings due to the high contrast between a white background and the circular gray grating patches[8]—was addressed[9] and implemented by creating the grating patch edges, which are smoothed into a gray background (the average of the grating patches). Other improvements of the FACT over the VCTS included equal 0.15 log-unit contrast

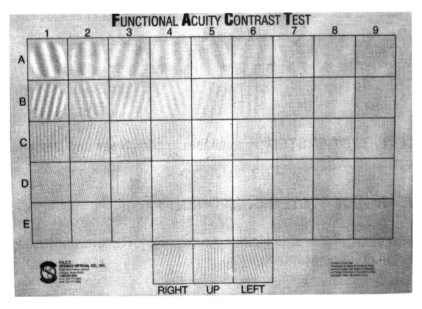

FIGURE 5-1 The Functional Acuity Contrast Test (FACT).

steps for greater sensitivity to contrast change, a larger patch size to test larger retinal areas, and digitally produced gratings for higher-quality sine waves.

After the sine-wave grating charts were introduced, several low-contrast letter charts were developed. The Regan chart[10] represented a simple approach, reducing the contrast of a standard Snellen-type letter acuity chart to several levels resulting in several charts. The Pelli-Robson chart[11] took a different approach and, on one chart, reduced a triplet of three letters in 0.15 log-unit contrast steps from high to low contrast. Although low-contrast acuity charts have been considered to be contrast sensitivity tests, they do not provide a contrast sensitivity curve or function similar to that of sine-wave contrast sensitivity charts. Indeed, as Leguire[12] has pointed out, there are important differences between sine-wave grating and low-contrast letter acuity charts.

One example of the confusion surrounding measurement of contrast sensitivity versus low-contrast letters is using the high "reliability" of 0.98 on the Pelli-Robson low-contrast letter acuity chart as a "standard."[11] Although low-contrast letter acuity charts may obtain high test-retest reliability, their sensitivity to important contrast losses may be low (e.g., to early cataract, as will be discussed later). Rubin[13] found the test-retest reliability of a computer-based sine-wave grating system using a forced-choice procedure to be 0.77. The grating contrast tests have also been reported within that range by Leguire,[12] who found VCTS test-retest reliabilities averaging 0.78 across five spatial frequencies from children.

Since the early 1960s the sine qua non for using sine-wave contrast sensitivity has been to measure and describe the basic mechanisms of vision—channels. The visual channels of the retinal/brain system are discrete filters of a size and spatial frequency to create the fundamental building blocks of perception.[1] Sine-wave gratings have been used not only to map out the perceptual properties of channels but also to measure their sensitivity to contrast. It has been demonstrated that only sine-wave gratings can measure the elementary visual channel tuned to one spatial frequency at a particular orientation.

The sensitivity and specificity to visual mechanisms and the relevance to clinical and functional vision for gratings and letters can be easily compared simply by plotting the grating and letter spatial frequency, along with size and contrast sensitivity, on the same graph.[15] The contrast sensitivity curve has been the most widely accepted analytical tool for understanding and quantifying vision and visual mechanisms. Because low-contrast letter acuity test results are typically plotted in a different manner, comparison with grating contrast sensitivity is difficult. However, by using the general relationship of threshold letter identification requiring about 2 cycles per letter, the contrast sensitivity of gratings and letters or any target can be compared.[1]

The abscissa in Figure 5-2 shows the relationship between spatial frequency and Snellen acuity of letters. Snellen acuity, shown from 100

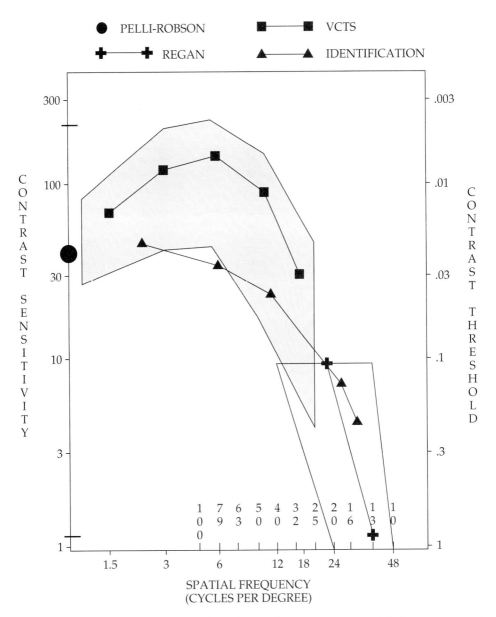

FIGURE 5-2 This chart shows the relationship between spatial frequency and Snellen acuity of letters.

to 10 located above the spatial frequency notation from 1.5 to 48, is the numerator of the usual "20/xx" notation. The ordinate shows the contrast threshold and contrast sensitivity of both gratings and letters. Plotted on this figure are the average contrast sensitivities of a sine-wave grating chart (the VCTS[9]), a single-size low-contrast letter chart (the Pelli-Robson chart,[11]), a multisize low-contrast letter chart system (the Regan charts[10]), and a curve of the identification contrast threshold for a Snellen letter chart.[7] The identification contrast threshold shows the upper limit of sensitivity that can be obtained using low contrast letters. The sensitivity of the letters fails to reach the sensitivity of the gratings. As readily seen, each contrast test measures a different range of spatial frequencies and contrast levels.

The VCTS tests contrast levels ranging from 0.3 to 0.0038 over a range of 1.5, 3, 6, 12, and 18 cycles per degree. The Pelli-Robson chart tests one size, 20/360 Snellen or 0.72 cycle per degree (at the manufacturer's suggested test distance) over a contrast range of 0.91 to 0.005. The Regan charts test four levels of contrast—0.96, 0.5, 0.25, and 0.11—over a Snellen range of 20/200 to 20/10, or about 5 to 48 cpd. Note that the grating chart test has the capability of testing almost 30 times more contrast sensitivity at the peak (6 cpd) than the Regan chart has. At 18 cpd the grating chart is about 3 times more sensitive to contrast than the letter charts.

It is interesting to note that the three contrast tests measure basically three ranges of spatial frequency or size and, somewhat less differently, three ranges of contrast. This is seen in noting the average population norms of each test in Figure 5-2. The Pelli-Robson chart tests very low spatial frequencies or large sizes over 4 to 8 times larger than the region of peak sensitivity at 3 to 6 cycles per degree. The VCTS, SWCT, and FACT all test an approximately equal range of spatial frequencies around the peak frequencies. The Regan charts test spatial frequencies from peak and higher (although with less sensitivity). Note that the Regan normal population space (the open trapezoid) is generally a continuation of the VCTS normal population space (the shaded area), showing the utility of this approach.

Even after the VCTS, SWCT, and FACT are graphed on the same spatial frequency and contrast test space, it may be difficult for the lay person to translate these test spaces into everyday visual experience. However, when the street scene in Figure 5-3, *A,* is spatially filtered using the full spatial frequency ranges of the three tests shown in Figure 5-2, the resulting filtered images allow a direct comparison with the original-image size and contrast information being tested.

The results of such filtering are shown in the VCTS, SWCT, FACT, Pelli-Robson, and Regan images of Figure 5-3, *B* to *D.* (It is difficult to know what range of spatial frequencies the Pelli-Robson chart tests because letter identification depends upon the relevant letter spatial frequencies reaching threshold, which can vary considerably from one person to another. Therefore, a generous range [0.0 to 3 cpd] was used for the Pelli-Robson filtering.)

The Pelli-Robson chart is testing a size too large to be relevant to the scene in Figure 5-3, *B.* It may be useful for predicting the threshold visibility of large trucks in the fog but not for determining the presence

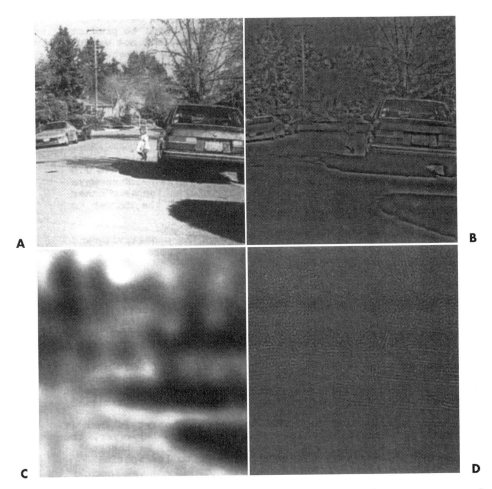

FIGURE 5-3 A, Spatially filtered street scene using full spatial frequency ranges of the three tests shown in figure 5-2; **B,** The Pelli-Robson chart is testing a size too large to be relevant to this scene; **C,** The VCTS tests a size and contrast range relevant to the complete scene information, especially the little girl; **D,** The Regan charts test the contrast and size range most relevant to the sharp edges of the scene which reveals little of the image quality and the little girl.

of small objects such as the little girl in the street. The VCTS tests a size and contrast range relevant to the complete scene information, especially the little girl in Figure 5-3, C. The Regan charts test the contrast and size range most relevant to the sharp edges of the scene, which reveals little of the image quality and the little girl (Fig. 5-3, D). The grating chart obtains and measures the most relevant information for evaluating one's ability to view this scene clearly.

At 30 mph, under normal weather and visibility conditions, the critical stopping sight distance is 158 feet from the little girl. A driver would have 2.5 seconds to see and avoid hitting the little girl. Sine-wave grating technology will provide the relevant information as to whether or not there is sufficient contrast sensitivity for the driver to see the girl in time to stop safely.

Understanding the important differences between the sensitivity and specificity of sine-wave gratings and the low-contrast letter acuity to measure contrast sensitivity in a clinically meaningful manner is exemplified by analysis of a recent paper on early cataract by Adamsons et al.[16]

The sine-wave grating test provided statistically significant losses from any type of early cataract at the higher spatial frequencies (12 and 18 cpd, as proven from other previous research). However, the Pelli-Robson low-contrast letter acuity test showed similar contrast between cataract and clear lenses, with the singular exception of posterior subcapsular cataracts. In addition, the Pelli-Robson chart results showed that the average cortical and nuclear cataract had *higher* contrast sensitivity than the clear lens. Clearly, the Pelli-Robson chart provides questionable contrast measures of early cataract and may underestimate their contrast loss.

Although Figures 3 and 4 of the Adamsons et al. paper[16] imply similar contrast sensitivity measurements, the way they are graphed, Figure 2 demonstrates why the grating chart but not the Pelli-Robson chart is able to detect contrast loss due to early cataract. Early cataract results in contrast loss primarily at the higher spatial frequencies, and gratings measuring contrast loss at higher frequencies can detect that loss. Because the Pelli-Robson chart measures very low spatial frequencies (0.72 cpd, which is 16.7 times larger size than the significant 12 cpd grating contrast losses reported by Adamsons et al.[16] detection of cataract in the early stages is not possible).

One commonly cited advantage of the Pelli-Robson chart is that it has high reliability relative to grating charts. However, the Adamsons et al. paper[16] shows that that advantage is moot, since the Pelli-Robson chart limits contrast loss measurement to low spatial frequencies and shows higher contrast loss from the clear lens compared with cortical and unclear cataract.

The opinion that the grating charts have poor reliability has been voiced by Rubin.[13] He used only one grating chart in his study rather than the three available that provide repeated measures and allow for determining means and standard deviations. This process provides a more statistically powerful measure than the Pelli-Robson two-of-three-letters-correct rule.[14] Many other reports have found the grating charts to be highly reliable (e.g., Leguire's research on amblyopia[12]).

Recently Ravalico et al.,[18] repeating Rubin's research, compared the grating and Pelli-Robson charts to visually evoked potentials (VEPs), a more objective measure of visual function. Replication of the previous results (i.e., low reliability of the grating chart) did not occur. They did, however, find that the grating chart measures were repeatable and, unlike the Pelli-Robson results, correlated with the VEPs.

Pelli et al.[11] and Rubin and Legge[19] have reported that the Pelli-Robson chart measures the peak of the grating contrast sensitivity curve. When the peak measure was used with a standard acuity measure, the parabolic curve could be plotted to determine a contrast sensitivity function.[16] Rohaly and Owsley[17] have demonstrated why both reports contain errors.

The Pelli-Robson chart is not an adequate predictor of peak contrast sensitivity, and the contrast sensitivity curve cannot be described by a single parametric curve. The inability of the Pelli-Robson chart to measure peak spatial frequencies and to be used as one of two free parameters to determine contrast sensitivity functions is easily explained by considering the variability of contrast sensitivity functions of normal observers.[6,7]

Also, the inability of any large letter or edge contrast tests to meaningfully measure contrast loss at the higher spatial frequencies or to be reliable at the peak frequencies should caution against their use in other contrast test applications of optical devices, drugs, or clinical conditions.

Test Modalities for Contrast Sensitivity

Contrast sensitivity testing can be accomplished with a chart, a lightbox, a view-in tester or a computer/video system. However, only the sine-wave test systems will be discussed here because of the inherent limitations and unknown clinical and functional utility of the other contrast test targets (e.g., letters) as discussed above. This is not to suggest that there may not be any use for other test targets for contrast sensitivity. However, little evidence exists for other test targets providing the breadth of contrast sensitivity information obtainable with gratings.

The VCTS, SWCT, and FACT charts test both near and far contrast sensitivity using an accompanying light meter to standardize light levels. By standardizing light levels for these test charts, it is possible to standardize contrast sensitivities, an important consideration not found in some light boxes. The advantages of the test charts are their low cost, simplicity, swiftness, and (for the near tests) portability and convenience. The disadvantages are their requirement for standardized room light levels and multiple charts for repeated measures.

The CVS-1000 (made by VectorVision) uses gratings in a "standardized" light box. Unfortunately, by standardizing the background light to room light level, it does not standardize the contrast. Rather, it standardizes the light level of the grating background surround. But the manner in which it does this allows the grating contrast to change. If the CVS-1000 is used in different lighting environments, the contrast of the test gratings will change.

For other evaluations it has been determined that the contrast changes for the VectorVision A1 and A4 gratings were 44% and 18% respectively from a dark room to a room with average luminance. The overall change in luminance across all grating patches was 13.3%. The individual grating patch luminances ranged from 7.9 to 12.8 ft-l under lights-off and from 10 to 14.8 ft-l under lights-on conditions. Thus, the room light level still must be standardized to standardize the CVS-1000.

An additional VectorVision product defect is that the variable white background of the CVS-1000 light box creates a source of glare. As room luminance decreases, the white background of the grating patches increases relative to the dark gray grating patches. Although the light into the eye from the white background remains constant, there is considerable contrast difference between the white background and the grating patch and this creates a glare source that is readily noticeable even in terms of afterimages.

The effect of increased glare is easily demonstrated by measuring the contrast sensitivity limit at row c with and without some haze material and with and without room lights. Whether or not this glare increases other problems such as aliased gratings[18] that can cause test errors, remains an open question.

Sine-wave grating contrast sensitivity is available in two view-in systems: the Multivision Contrast Tester (MCT, Vistech Consultants) and the OPTEC series (Stereo Optical). The MCT has the VCTS gratings under variable-controlled luminance with glare. The OPTECs have the SWCT and FACT gratings under controlled luminance and with glare option.

The main advantages of the view-in testers are that they eliminate the need to control room light levels and they require a small test space. With some of the OPTEC systems having other vision tests (e.g., color and stereopsis) these view-in systems offer considerable advantages. The main disadvantage is their increased expense over that of the charts if only contrast sensitivity testing is desired.

The computer/video grating tests—Optronix, BVAT, VisioWorks and VSG2/2—offer the highest degree of test flexibility in terms of technique, target configuration, and spatial frequencies. However, these systems are relatively costly and complex as well as require careful consideration and monitoring of contrast calibration of the video display.

Interpreting Contrast Sensitivity: EyeView

Scores obtained from testing vision with sine-wave gratings are graphed in a format which creates a contrast sensitivity curve as shown in Figure 5-2. Although the ability to interpret the shapes this curve can form comes with experience, it can be difficult to translate those shapes into meaningful descriptions for others. A recently developed tool that demonstrates the functional vision consequences of the contrast sensitivity curve are the pictures processed by EyeView™ (Visumetrics Corporation).

EyeView is an image-processing software program that creates either newspaper or street scene pictures modified by acuity or sine-wave grating contrast sensitivity data. When an EyeView-processed picture is compared with age-matched norms, acuity or contrast sensitivity, or pre- and post-treatment, the implications on seeing become readily apparent. EyeView allows others to "see" through the eyes of the patient.

A functionally important example of EyeView-processed pictures is demonstrated by a person with histoplasmosis. This person ran into an overturned truck on a major highway on a rainy night. Although tested at 20/25 acuity, her contrast sensitivity compared with that of an age-matched normal shown in Figure 5-4 is severely depressed at the low and especially so at the middle spatial frequencies. However, the high spatial frequencies are spared, resulting in her maintaining good acuity.

The EyeView-processed pictures show the severe consequences of her loss of contrast sensitivity. While the 20/25 acuity suggests good visual capability, the contrast sensitivity curve demonstrates otherwise. Note that the detail in the low-contrast picture is just as sharp as that in the 20/25 picture. This person has not lost the ability to see high-contrast detail, as evidenced by her 20/25 acuity. However, her loss of contrast of that detail as well as all the other picture information is her functional vision problem. Whereas the 20/25 picture could allow a large reduction in contrast before it looked similar to the low-contrast picture, a similar reduction in contrast of the low-contrast picture would render it unintelligible, virtually blank. Thus, the 20/25 picture would suggest that the person has a large contrast reserve while the low-contrast sensitivity person has little. Although it can never be proven that this poor vision was the sole cause of the accident, clearly this person would be visually handicapped under poor-contrast conditions such as on a rural highway on a rainy night.

In summary, the differences between contrast and spatial frequency and target size of any contrast tests are easily examined by plotting the average and normal population test spaces on the same graph, depicting contrast thresholds and spatial frequencies as well as size. This graphical form should become the standard by which test comparisons are performed. The filtered image technique then might be employed to demonstrate the relative importance of different test spaces to the visibility of real-world scenes and objects. Different test instruments for contrast sensitivity have different advantages and disadvantages. Finally, EyeView pictures allow one to begin to "see" the world through the eyes of the patient.

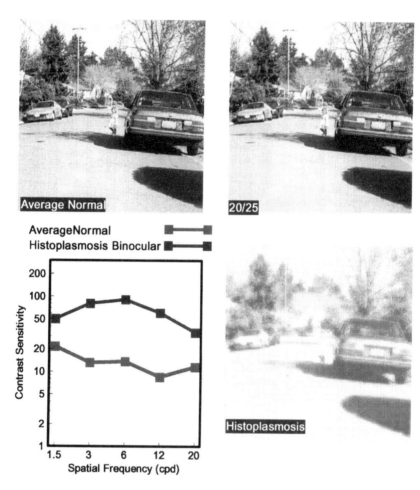

FIGURE 5-4 A street scene is shown with average/normal vision, 20/25 vision and histoplasmosis. The chart graphs contrast sensitivity and spatial frequency for average/normal vision and histoplasmosis binocular vision.

References

1. Ginsburg AP: Spatial filtering and visual form perception. In Boff K (ed): *Handbook of perception and human performance*, New York, 1986, John Wiley & Sons, vol 2, pp 34-41.
2. Owsley C, Sloane M: Contrast sensitivity, acuity, and the perception of "real world" targets, *Br J Ophthalmol* 71:791-796, 1987.
3. Decina LE, Staplin L: Retrospective evaluation of alternative vision screening criteria for older and younger drivers, *Accid Anal Prev* 25:267-275, 1993.
4. Ginsburg AP, Rosenthal B, Cohen J: The evaluation of reading capability of low vision patients using the Vision Contrast Test System (VCTS). In Woo GC (ed): *Low vision: principles and applications*, New York, 1987, Springer-Verlag, pp 17-28.
5. Faye EE: Low vision management in selected eye diseases. In Woo GC (ed): *Low vision: principles and applications*, New York, 1987, Springer-Verlag, pp 96-107.

6. Arden GB, Jacobson JJ: A simple grating test for contrast sensitivity: preliminary results indicate value in screening for glaucoma, *Invest Ophthalmol Vis Sci* 17:23-32, 1978.
7. Ginsburg AP: Clinical findings from a new contrast sensitivity test chart. In Fiorentini A, Guyton DL, Siegel IM (eds): *Advances in diagnostic visual optics*, New York, 1987, Springer-Verlag, pp 132-140.
8. Thorn F: Effects of dioptric blur on the Vistech contrast sensitivity test, *Optom Vis Sci* 57:8-12, 1990.
9. Ginsburg AP: Spatial frequency and contrast sensitivity test chart, U.S. Patent no. 4,365,873, 1982.
10. Regan, D, Neima D: Low-contrast letter charts as a test of visual functions, *Ophthalmology* 90:1192-1200, 1983.
11. Pelli DG, Robson JG, Wilkins AJ: The design of a new letter chart for measuring contrast sensitivity, *Clin Vis Sci* 2:187-199, 1988.
12. Leguire LE: Do letter charts measure contrast sensitivity? *Clin Vis Sci* 6:391-400, 1991.
13. Rubin G: Reliability and sensitivity of clinical contrast sensitivity tests, *Clin Vis Sci* 1:169-177, 1989.
14. Rogers GL, Bremer DL, Leguire LE: Contrast sensitivity functions in normal children with the Vistech method, *J Pediatr Ophthalmol Strabismus* 24:216-219, 1987.
15. Ginsburg AP: Testing functional vision: important relationships between grating contrast sensitivity and low-contrast letter acuity tests, *SPIE* 2127:36-43, 1994.
16. Adamsons I, Rubin G, Vitale S, et al.: The effect of early cataracts on glare and contrast sensitivity, *Arch Ophthalmol* 110:1081-1086, 1992.
17. Rohaly AM, Owsley C: Modeling the contrast sensitivity functions of older adults, *J Opt Soc Am* 10:1591-1599, 1993.
18. Ravalico G, Baccara F, Rinaldi G: Contrast sensitivity in multifocal intraocular lenses, *J Cataract Refract Surg* 19:22-25, 1993.
19. Rubin GS, Legge GE: The psychophysics of reading. VI. The role of contrast in low vision, *Vision Res* 29:79-91, 1989.

6

Visual Field Testing in the Low Vision Patient

Sherry J. Bass
Jerome Sherman

Key Terms

Automated perimetry   Optic nerve disease   Macular disease
Retinal degeneration

Some people say it's not what you see but how you see it. Although there are many ways to determine what a low vision patient sees, perimetry is one of the few testing methods that actually defines how and to what extent the low vision patient perceives his world.

Perimetry can be difficult in the best of circumstances, but field testing in the low vision patient requires more patience and challenges a practitioner's technical and interpretative skills more than any other aspect of vision management in disadvantaged populations. In addition to difficulty with concentrating and loss of visual sensitivity, the inability of some patients to maintain fixation may make threshold measurements invalid, time consuming (arduous), and unreliable.

Principles of Automated Perimetry

For a long time the standard in field testing of the low vision patient was Goldmann perimetry, which required a perimetrist to painstakingly plot out the visual field. Although this had certain advantages (the use of kinetic stimuli in the presentation, the constant presence of a perimetrist), manual perimetry lacked the standardization, and hence the ability to compare results, that could determine change. Moreover, the automated perimeter (unlike a manual perimetrist, who is aware of the pathology) does not have a preconceived notion as to what the resultant field should appear to be.

CLINICAL PEARL

Automated perimetry has paved the way for more standardized and accurate visual field testing in all types of patients, including those with low vision.

Automated perimetry has paved the way for more standardized and accurate visual field testing in all types of patients, including those with low vision. There are numerous features that facilitate visual field testing and remove any of the problems inherent in manual perimetry:

1. A variety of screening and threshold programs designed to provide the maximum information in the shortest possible time
2. The ability to determine thresholds without a perimetrist, which removes bias and improves both validity and reliability
3. Better methods of monitoring fixation and determining patient variability factors
4. Larger, and in some cases kinetic, fixation targets for better concentration and more accurate fixation
5. The ability to numerically determine threshold levels for statistical analyses and comparative purposes

Some perimeters—such as the Dicon TKS 4000 and the LD 400 (see color plate 1, *A, B*) offer moving fixation targets (of standard and large size), multiple stimuli, and computerized voices to help maintain patient attention and concentration. Others—like the Octopus 1-2-3 (manufactured by Interzeag)—offer constant fixation control via a contrast monitor and camera. If the patient looks away from fixation, the contrast monitor detects a difference in contrast between the pupil and iris and automatically rejects the data. The Humphrey field analyzer provides both a small and a large diamond for low vision patients with a central scotoma.

Automated perimeters are set up to automatically run a specified program for measuring the visual field. They construct a specific "hill

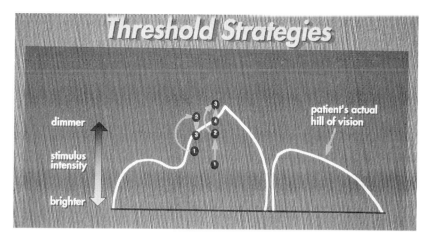

FIGURE 6-1 Automated perimeters determine a patient's hill of vision based on central threshold values and then test around that threshold. (Courtesy Humphrey Instruments, Inc.)

of vision" by presenting static stimuli within the central 5° to determine the patient's central threshold. The other points in the field are tested based on these central values. Consistent with the hill of vision, the further from fixation the perimeter presents the stimuli the brighter they become; thus a normal patient is able to see them (Fig. 6-1). Most perimeters then compare the patient's visual field with the fields of other patients of the same age and without ocular disease.

The perimeter can run *screening* programs, to determine if there is a diseased eye, or *threshold* programs, to quantify the extent of disease in the eye. In a screening program, which can generally take from 3 to 6 minutes to perform (but may take longer), stimuli are presented in a static mode at a level 6 decibels (db) above the patient's central threshold. If the patient sees them, his response is often recorded as a check or a circle. If he does not see them, this may be recorded as a triangle or a black square (Fig. 6-2).

In some screening programs the perimeter determines the threshold values for the points missed.

In threshold programs, a threshold value is determined for each point tested. This value is the stimulus intensity that is seen one out of every two times it is presented (the so-called 50% probability-of-seeing curve). Threshold values, in decibels, lend themselves to statistical analyses and comparisons. Changes in the patient's visual field are more readily apparent when numbers are used as opposed to pictures. Threshold visual fields can be presented with (1) the actual threshold numbers, (2) the difference between the patient's threshold values and those of a disease-free same-aged individual, or (3) a gray scale in

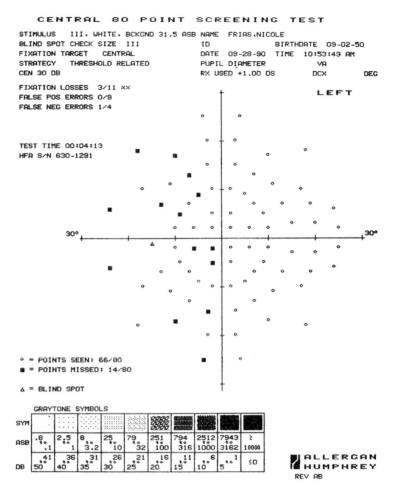

FIGURE 6-2 Results of a central 80 point screening test on the Humphrey visual field analyzer. Points not seen at 6 db above central threshold are depicted as *black squares*. (Courtesy Humphrey Instruments, Inc.)

CLINICAL PEARL

Threshold values, in decibels, lend themselves to statistical analyses and comparisons. Changes in the patient's visual field are more readily apparent when numbers are used as opposed to pictures.

which existent data are extrapolated to fill in the areas not tested (Fig. 6-3). Some perimeters can also present the data, both screening and threshold, in a three-dimensional format that depicts the patient's actual hill of vision based on the testing results (see color plate 2).

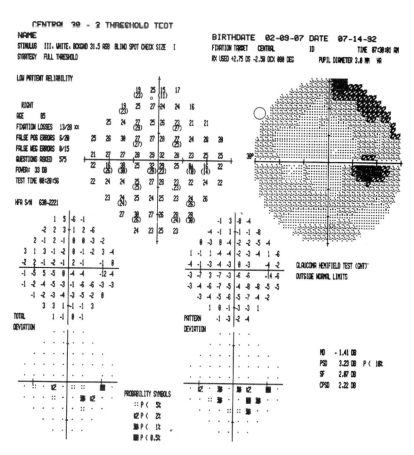

FIGURE 6-3 Results of a central 30-2 threshold program on the Humphrey visual field analyzer are depicted in gray scale as well as in absolute threshold value and difference value scales. (Courtesy Humphrey Instruments, Inc.)

Because they already have an eye that is diseased, most low vision patients will require a threshold visual field program. The question remains: How much is the ocular disease affecting visual function in the low vision patient? Low vision patients with diffuse retinal disease or advanced glaucoma may require a larger testing stimulus (e.g., the Goldmann V target) if they have significantly reduced acuity. Those with macular degeneration or optic nerve disease resulting in a large central scotoma may require a larger fixation target instead of the standard spot or light. However, once nonstandard testing parameters are used, statistical analysis of the data is no longer possible on most systems. This is because most perimeters performing statistical data analysis base their output on data procured from normals using standard testing parameters.

Eventually, some of these perimeters will have enough of a data base using nonstandard targets to perform statistical analyses of the data under all testing conditions.

Interpretation of Visual Field Results

Whereas automated perimetry makes it relatively easy to perform visual field testing, the interpretation still lies with the practitioner. Many automated programs include statistical packages to perform quite sophisticated data analyses, which present the practitioner with a statement or report about whether the data lie inside or outside normal limits compared to those for a same-aged disease-free population. This certainly helps with interpretation, but the decision concerning the significance of abnormal findings, at least at the present level of automated perimetry, remains a clinical one to be determined by a human being and not a machine.

CLINICAL PEARL

Whereas automated perimetry makes it relatively easy to perform visual field testing, the interpretation still lies with the practitioner.

Interpretation of automated perimetry findings in the low vision patient can best be discussed by presentation of interesting and unique retinal and optic nerve head anomalies and pathologies, both acquired and inherited, that result in reduced visual function.

Case One

An asymptomatic 39-year-old white pharmacist was referred for further evaluation following a routine eye examination that had revealed decreased visual acuity with no obvious pathology. The referring optometrist performed threshold visual field testing and obtained a ring scotoma around fixation that he could not explain; he therefore sent the patient for additional testing. No visual problems whatsoever were reported, including no nyctalopia. Entering best-corrected visual acuities were 20/30+2 OU. Examination of the fundi revealed slightly attenuated arterioles and peripapillary pigment rings OU. No pigmentary changes were noted anywhere else in either fundus (see color plate 3). The testing was done with a Dicon TKS 4000 120-point Quantify Missed Points (QMP) program, which revealed paracentral scotomas but essentially normal mid- and far-peripheral fields (see color plate 4). The referring practitioner thought this patient was malingering or producing a "hysterical" visual field. However, the Dicon automated perimeter (which uses a kinetic fixation point) virtually eliminated that possibility. These fields closely matched the fields from the referring doctor, who had used a Humphrey automated perimeter.

Because of the abnormal fields and the presence of slightly attenuated arterioles, electroretinography was performed. The responses under photopic conditions were reduced by about two thirds, and under scotopic conditions by about half. Based on these findings, the patient clearly had a diffuse retinal disease, which in this case was classified as a mild form of atypical inverse retinitis pigmentosa sine pigmento. With only slightly reduced visual acuity and paracentral field defects, he was told he had cone-rod degeneration, as opposed to the rod-cone form of this disease. The visual field findings were ring scotomas, an early field defect in retinitis pigmentosa, but because of his age and asymptomatic state, with reduced ERGs, it was decided he had a mild form of the disease. He claimed to have no family history of this condition.

Although manual perimetry might have yielded similar fields, automated perimetry allowed for helpful diagnostic software applications that enabled both the patient and the doctor to appreciate the field defect from a three-dimensional point of view. The patient was educated about his condition and is currently being followed. He is also arranging to have his siblings and children examined.

Case Two

A 25-year-old woman who worked as an artist in the textile industry presented with complaints that objects appeared to jump around. She had a sister who had been diagnosed with Stargardt's disease (hereditary macular degeneration), and she wanted to know if she had a similar condition. Best corrected visual acuities were 20/50 OD and 20/40 OS. Internal examination of the eyes revealed normal optic nerve heads and fundi. Examination of the maculas revealed foveal reflexes with subtle pigment mottling (see color plate 5). Visual field testing with Goldmann manual perimetry did not reveal any abnormalities. Visual evoked potentials were reduced in amplitude but normal in latency. Fluorescein angiography was recommended to further elucidate any macular abnormalities, but the patient refused. Based on her family history and the subtle macular abnormalities, a diagnosis of Stargardt's macular degeneration was made.

During subsequent follow-up examination, the patient complained of progressively deteriorating vision. At her last examination, best corrected visual acuities had dropped to 20/200 OU. Visual field testing with the Dicon automated central 10° threshold program revealed a central scotoma in each eye displaced superiorly because of the slight eccentric fixation (see color plate 6). Ophthalmoscopy now revealed subtle retinal pigment epithelial changes in each macula along with some yellowish flecks. The visual field defects in this case were far more indicative of the patient's reduced visual function than the ophthalmoscopic picture would have led one to believe. A central 10° threshold program often provides more information than a 30° program regarding field loss due to macular disease because it tests points approximately 2° apart as opposed to 6° apart. In cases such as this, in which the funduscopic picture may not be diagnostic, 10° threshold fields are extremely useful.

CLINICAL PEARL

The visual field defects in early Stargardt's disease were far more indicative of the patient's reduced visual function than the ophthalmoscopic picture would have led one to believe.

Case Three

A 42-year-old Hispanic taxi driver presented for an eye examination complaining of blur in his left eye over the preceding 3 months. Best corrected visual acuities were 20/20 OD and 20/100 OS. External examination revealed a 1+ afferent pupillary defect OS. Internal examination disclosed normal optic nerveheads, maculas, and fundi. Amsler grid testing showed temporal field loss OS but not OD. More in-depth field testing with the Humphrey field analyzer central threshold 30-2 program revealed a temporal hemianopsia OS that respected the midline as well as a superotemporal defect OD (Fig. 6-4). Because of the loss of vision and the bitemporal field defect, he was referred for imaging studies. CT scanning indicated the presence of a 3 cm pituitary adenoma (Fig. 6-5), and subsequent MRI confirmed that it was actually 6 cm. This case demonstrates the importance of performing visual field testing in *both* eyes in any patient complaining of a loss of vision even in *one* eye. A field defect in the "normal" eye can signal the presence of a visual pathway lesion that requires neuroimaging studies.

CLINICAL PEARL

A field defect in the "normal" eye of a patient complaining of monocular visual acuity loss can signal the presence of a visual pathway lesion that requires neuroimaging studies.

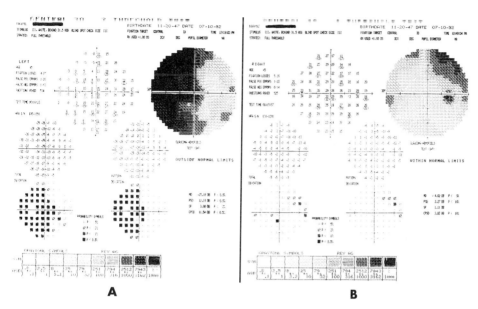

FIGURE 6-4 Case 3: A central 30-2 threshold program reveals, **A**, a temporal hemianopsia in the left eye that respects the midline and, **B**, a superotemporal defect in the right eye.

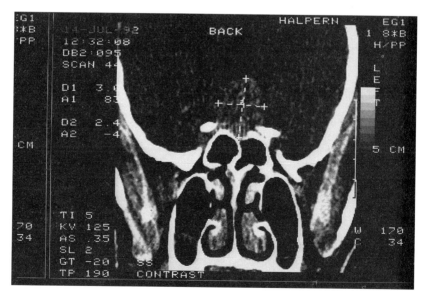

FIGURE 6-5 Case 3: A 3 cm pituitary adenoma by CT was later found to be 6 cm by MRI.

Case Four

A 58-year-old black woman presented with a history of high myopia and an old retinal detachment in her left eye that had not progressed or been treated. Her best corrected visual acuities were 20/40 OU. Internal examination OS revealed lattice degeneration superiorly and an old inferior retinal detachment with a densely pigmented demarcation band (see color plate 7). Examination OD showed multiple areas of lattice degeneration with atrophic holes (some with vitreal strands attached) and an inferotemporal retinal schisis. Visual fields testing with a 0-60 threshold program revealed an absolute superior field defect OS corresponding to the old inferior retinal detachment (see color plate 8). Since the detachment extended about 10° below the disc, one could predict that the corresponding field defect would extent to within 10° of the blind spot superiorly.

An old or relatively old untreated retinal detachment will cause a visual field defect because the retina is no longer functional in the area that has been detached. The presence of the demarcation band posterior to the detachment seals the retina in the area and helps prevent additional progression of the detachment. A retinoschisis will also cause a visual field defect, because in this condition there is a splitting of the retina at the outer plexiform layer (acquired retinoschisis) or the nerve fiber layer (congenital). Therefore, although retinoschisis is not a detachment, the visual signals or impulses cannot travel to the optic nerve and there is thus a corresponding absolute visual field defect.

Case Five

A 42-year-old white computer programmer with a history of high myopia and 20/20 acuity OU presented for an eye examination complaining of a 1-day history of constant blurring in the lower corner of his right eye. The initial examiner had noticed a superior retinal abnormality but failed to recognize it as a detachment. Referral to a retinal specialist was delayed for 5 days, by which time the detachment had progressed to involve the posterior pole, with a subsequent reduction in acuity to 20/200.

The retina was successfully reattached by cryopexy with a scleral buckle, but the patient still had distortions, micropsia, and a loss of peripheral vision OD with best corrected acuity 20/50. Visual field testing using a 0-60 program showed relative peripheral field depression in all four quadrants (see color plate 9). In total there was a 42% loss of retinal sensitivity in the periphery of the right eye compared to the left, which was likely due to the delay in receiving treatment and resulted in a larger retinal detachment, necessitating the scleral buckle.

Additionally, the retina was detached for a longer time, and this increased the likelihood of irreversible functional loss. The patient sued the initial examining doctor for failure to make a more prompt referral, and the case is still pending. Visual field testing in this patient was a useful adjunct in the documentation of peripheral vision loss.

Case Six

A 23-year-old black athletic instructor presented with complaints of bilaterally reduced vision over the preceding month and headaches that sometimes woke him up. His only known health history was a problem with one knee. Best corrected visual acuities were 20/40 OD and 20/30 OS. All aspects of the initial eye examination, including the fundi (see color Plate 10), were normal. However, the patient did not manifest any responses to pattern visual evoked potentials, indicating a visual pathway problem. MRI showed evidence of periventricular "hotspots," which suggested a demyelinating process, but bilateral hilar adenopathy at chest x-ray was indicative of sarcoidosis. His vision began dropping, and a regimen of 60 mg prednisone was started. One month later his vision had dropped to 20/400 OD but was still 20/30 OS. Temporal pallor of both optic nerves was evident (see color plate 11). Visual field testing OD with a 30-degree program revealed central field loss (Fig. 6-6, A). Testing OS showed a denser central field loss (Fig. 6-6, B). Despite continued use of the steroids, his vision failed to improve and the fields remained stable.

In the absence of macular disease, central scotomas are indicative of optic nerve disease. This patient had CNS sarcoidosis with transneuronal degeneration, which explained why the optic nerveheads had developed temporal pallor after the initial visit. Visual fields were helpful in suggesting an optic neuropathy in this patient. Although his vision did not improve, he fared better than most do with neurosarcoidosis, probably because of the timely initiation of steroid therapy.

Case Seven

A 74-year-old retired highschool principal with a history of chronic open angle glaucoma presented with a new complaint, a "blind spot" to the right of fixation when reading. An old retinal detachment in the left eye led to his using the right eye only. A 30° field did not reveal any defect that could explain his complaint (see color plate 12, A). A 10° field showed a 6° relative scotoma to the right of fixation that corresponded to his chief complaint (see color plate 12, B).

Monocular patients frequently are more aware of relative field defects than binocular patients are. A scotoma immediately to the right

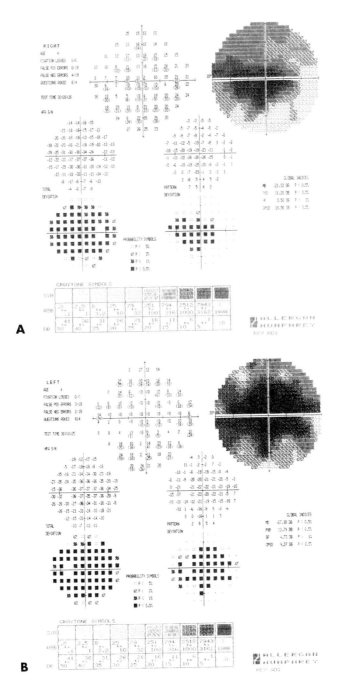

FIGURE 6-6 Case 6: Visual field testing OD with a central 30° threshold program reveals central field loss, **A**, but denser central loss OS, **B**.

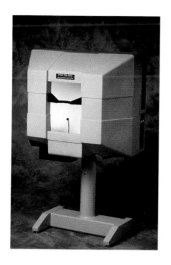

A

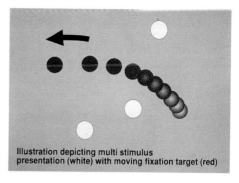

Illustration depicting multi stimulus presentation (white) with moving fixation target (red)

B

PLATE 1 **A**, The Dicon TKS 4000 automated perimeter. **B**, A moving fixation target maintains attention. (Courtesy Dicon/Vismed, Inc.)

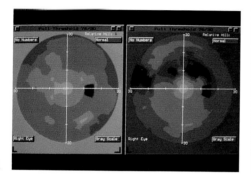

A

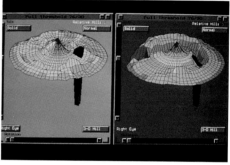

B

PLATE 2 **A**, Results of the central 30° threshold program on the Dicon TKS 4000 presentation of an initially normal field with subsequent glaucomatous change (Bjerrum scotoma), depicted as a gray scale. **B**, Same fields with the three-dimensional hill of vision presentation showing erosion in the superior part of the hill (Bjerrum scotoma). (Courtesy Dicon/Vismed, Inc.)

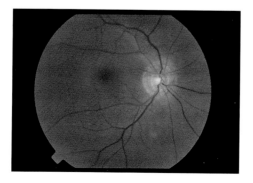

PLATE 3 Case 1: Slightly attenuated arterioles and peripapillary pigment rings (fundus photograph).

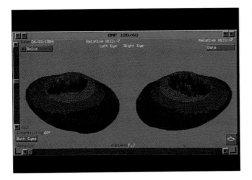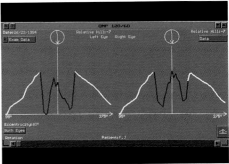

PLATE 4   Case 1: Visual field testing reveals paracentral scotomas but essentially normal mid- and far-peripheral fields.

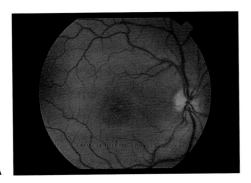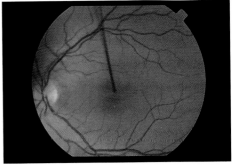

A   **B**

PLATE 5   Case 2: The maculas in this Stargardt patient display foveal reflexes with only subtle pigment mottling. Visual acuities were 20/50 OD, **A**, and 20/40 OS, **B**. Note that the patient fixates with the superior part of her fovea because the inferior half is not functional. This translates into the superior field defect seen in Plate 6.

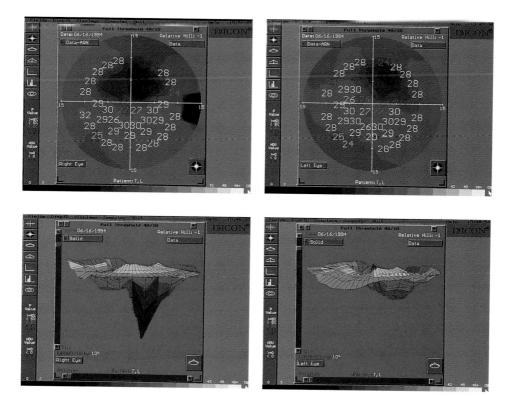

PLATE 6 Case 2: Visual field testing at a later date with a central 10° threshold program. Visual acuities had dropped to 20/200 OU. Central scotomas in each eye are displaced superiorly because of eccentric fixation.

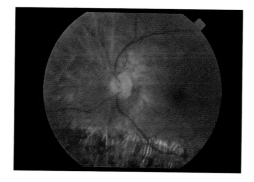

PLATE 7 Case 4: An old inferior retinal detachment with a densely pigmented demarcation band.

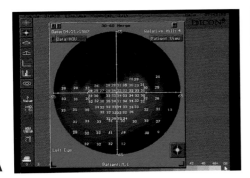

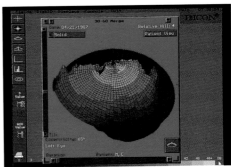

A

B

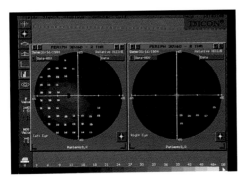

C

PLATE 8 Case 4: Visual field testing using a 0-60 threshold program revealed an absolute superior field defect corresponding to the inferior retinal detachment. **A**, Gray scale; **B**, three-dimensional hill of vision; **C**, isopter plot.

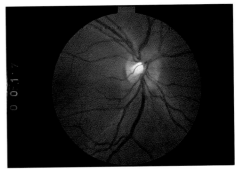

PLATE 9 Case 5: Visual field testing using a 0-60 threshold program revealed relative field depression in all four quadrants OD compared to OS.

PLATE 10 Case 6: Normal fundus of a patient with reduced acuity (OD).

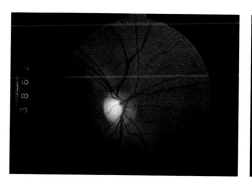 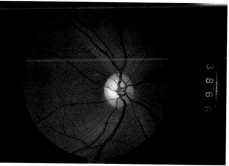

A **B**

PLATE 11 Case 6: One month later, temporal pallor of both optic nerves is evident. **A**, OD; **B**, OS.

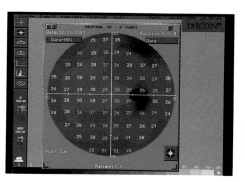 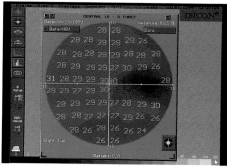

A **B**

PLATE 12 Case 7: Visual field testing with a central 30° threshold program fails to reveal any field defects, **A**, but with a central 10° program reveals a 6° relative scotoma to the right of fixation, **B**. This corresponded to the patient's chief complaint.

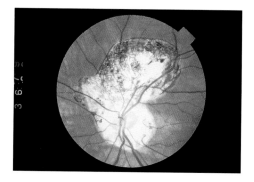

PLATE 13 Case 8: Inactive toxoplasmosis lesion superior to and contiguous with the disc (fundus photograph).

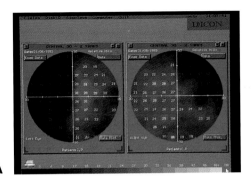 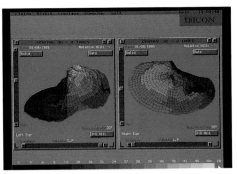

A   B

PLATE 14 Cast 9: Visual field testing reveals a bitemporal hemianopsia with 20/20 acuity. **A**, Gray scale; **B**, three-dimensional hill.

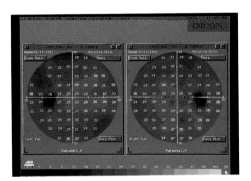 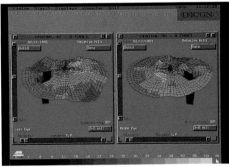

A₁   A₂

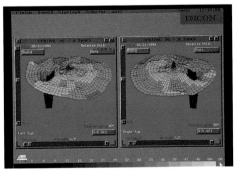

B₁   B₂

PLATE 15 Case 9: Visual fields 1 month after surgery, **A**, revealed a noticeable improvement compared to before surgery (**A₁** gray scale, **A₂** three-dimensional hill) and 9 months after surgery, **B**, continue to show improvement (**B₁** gray scale, **B₂** three-dimensional hill).

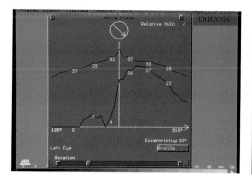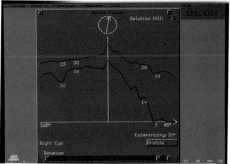

PLATE 16 Case 9: A delta or change program of meridional fields showing the significant improvement that can occur after surgery.

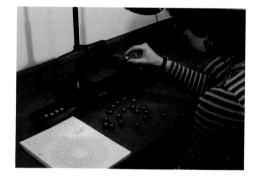

PLATE 17 A patient arranging one of the four boxes in the Farnsworth-Munsell 100-Hue Test.

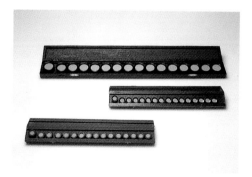

PLATE 18 Three versions of the Farnsworth Dichotomous Test for Color Blindness-Panel D-15. **Top to bottom:** A jumbo version produced by Ehrnst and Georgeson, the standard D-15 test, and a desaturated version produced by Adams.

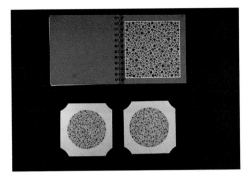

PLATE 19 Two examples of pseudoisochromatic plate (PIP) tests. **Top**: The AO-HRR plates; **bottom**: Ishihara's Tests for Colour Blindness.

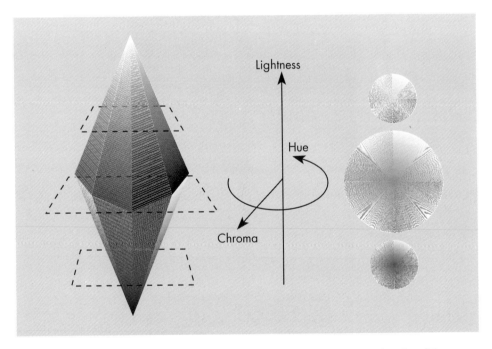

PLATE 20 Solid representation of the perceptual attributes of color. Hues are ordered on a closed dimension (shown here as circumferences of the solid). Shades of gray fall on the lightness axis and are called achromatic colors. Chroma is the horizontal distance from the lightness axis and represents the chromatic intensity of the color, independent of its lightness. The three color circles on the right represent slices through a colored solid taken at planes indicated by the dashed lines on the solid.

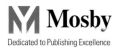
Mosby
Dedicated to Publishing Excellence

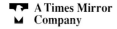
A Times Mirror
Company

ERRATA

Dear Customer:

Thank you for your interest in *Functional Assessment of Low Vision*, by Bruce P. Rosenthal, OD, FAAO and Roy G. Cole, OD, FAAO.

It has come to our attention that in Color Plates 20 and 21 in this book, the colors are incorrect. We encourage you to replace the incorrect plates with the enclosed corrected plates.

We hope that these errors will in no way diminish your confidence in this outstanding book; it was thoroughly reviewed for accuracy. Mosby prides itself on producing high quality educational materials for health–care professionals. We sincerely regret the errors and apologize for any inconvenience. As a publisher with a long tradition of publishing excellence, our goal is to continue to meet your needs for reliable educational materials.

Sincerely,

Don Ladig
Publisher

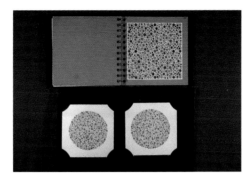

PLATE 19 Two examples of pseudoisochromatic plate (PIP) tests. **Top**: The AO-HRR plates; **bottom**: Ishihara's Tests for Colour Blindness.

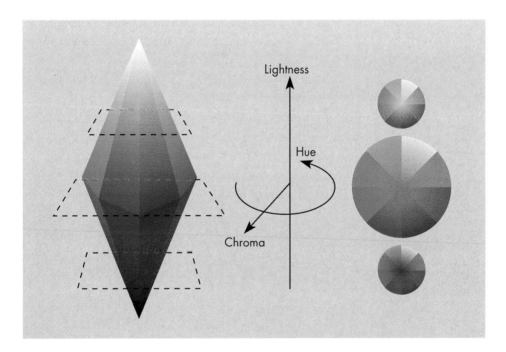

PLATE 20 Solid representation of the perceptual attributes of color. Hues are ordered on a closed dimension (shown here as circumferences of the solid). Shades of gray fall on the lightness axis and are called achromatic colors. Chroma is the horizontal distance from the lightness axis and represents the chromatic intensity of the color, independent of its lightness. The three color circles on the right represent slices through a colored solid taken at planes indicated by the dashed lines on the solid.

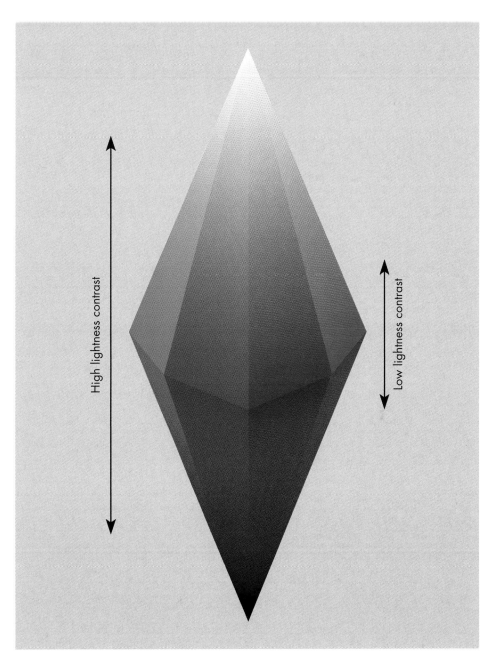

PLATE 21 Effective contrasts for patients with color deficits generally require using colors with very different lightnesses.

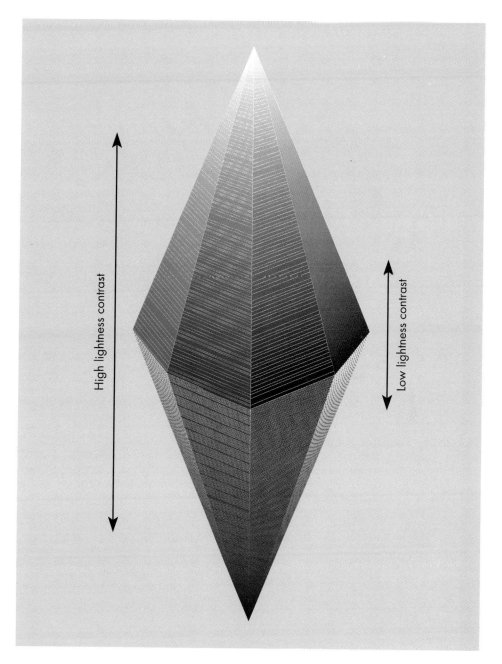

PLATE 21 Effective contrasts for patients with color deficits generally require using colors with very different lightnesses.

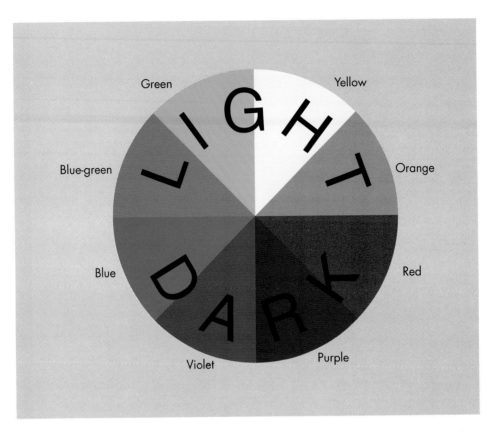

PLATE 22 This hue circle is arranged so the colors in its bottom half tend to appear darker to patients with color deficits than they do to people with normal color vision. To ensure that this effect does not reduce effective contrast for these people, select the dark colors in a contrast from the bottom half of the circle and light colors from the top half.

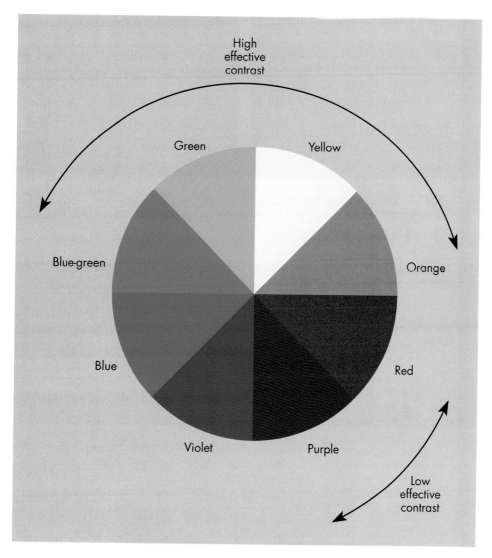

PLATE 23 Since patients with color deficits always have more difficulty distinguishing neighboring hues, contrast colors from very different rather than adjacent locations on the hue circle.

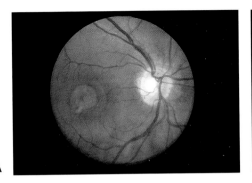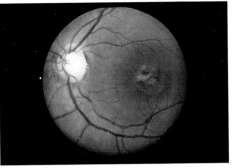

A

B

PLATE 24 **A**, The egg-yolk phase of Best's vitelleruptive dystrophy. **B**, The latter "scrambled-egg" phase in a different patient. This is associated with reduced visual acuity.

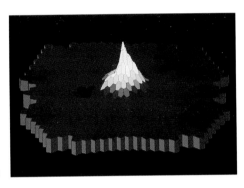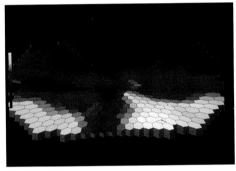

A

B

PLATE 25 **A**, Topographical ERG for the central 60° of a normal patient. The amplitude peak corresponds to the fovea and then declines gradually toward the periphery. **B**, Topographical ERG for a patient with no observable macular lesion. Visual acuity was 20/40–. Note the very reduced pattern from the macula.

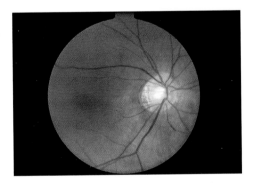

PLATE 26 A normal fundus of the patient in Case 4. Congenital nystagmus and flat ERGs supported the diagnosis of Leber's congenital amaurosis.

of fixation in a monocular patient often results in a complaint of losing one's place while reading. This Jewish patient, fluent in Hebrew, might have tried reading this right-to-left language and perhaps have been less troubled by his scotoma. Any patient with a complaint that appears to originate near the visual axis may require a 10° threshold field test.

CLINICAL PEARL

Any patient with a complaint that appears to originate near the visual axis may require a 10° threshold field test.

Case Eight

A 32-year-old white woman presented with the complaint that the lower part of her visual field was missing. Her right eye was "useless" because of a large congenital scar affecting the macula and surrounding the optic nervehead. She had recently been treated for a reactivation of toxoplasmosis of her left retina. Visual acuities were hand motion OD and 20/25 OS. The fundus lesion, now inactive, was superior to and contiguous with the disc (see color plate 13). The 60° field showed essentially no inferior half (Fig. 6-7).

Toxoplasma gondii is known to live encysted in the nerve fiber layer for up to 25 years, only to become reactivated and cause a retinochoroiditis and overlying vitritis. The nerve fiber layer is the primary site of reactivation and hence will be severely compromised. Since the ganglion cell axons immediately around the disc are densely packed, a relatively small lesion there can cause a much larger field defect. Although the photoreceptors are still functioning superior to the lesion, the ganglion cell axons are destroyed at the time of the reactivation. Thus there is a break in the neural chain conducting visual impulses to the brain. It is for this reason that both the size of the lesion and its location must be considered in predicting a field defect from a fundus lesion.

Case Nine

A 55-year-old woman presented with vague complaints of vision problems. She occasionally saw double but had recently noticed that a problem was present even when she had "single" vision. Best corrected visual acuity was 20/20 OU and the external and internal examinations were unremarkable. Visual fields disclosed a bitemporal hemianopsia

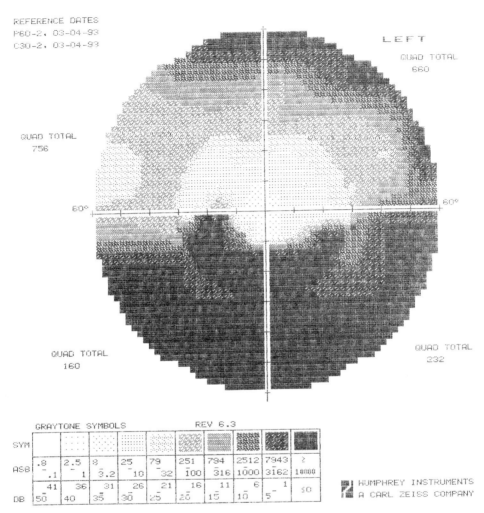

FIGURE 6-7 Case 8: A 0-60 visual field test reveals essentially no inferior field.

(see color plate 14). MRI revealed a chiasmal mass, which was surgically removed and identified as a pituitary adenoma (Fig. 6-8). Visual fields then showed an improvement compared to the fields before surgery (see color plate 15).

It is possible to repeat threshold visual fields under precisely the same conditions at a later date and appreciate the change that has occurred. The delta (or change) program of meridional fields in this patient before and after removal of the tumor showed remarkable field normalization (see color plate 16). Visual field improvements may be seen following tumor removal, after treatment of infections of the retina or brain, and even occasionally in chronic open angle glaucoma.

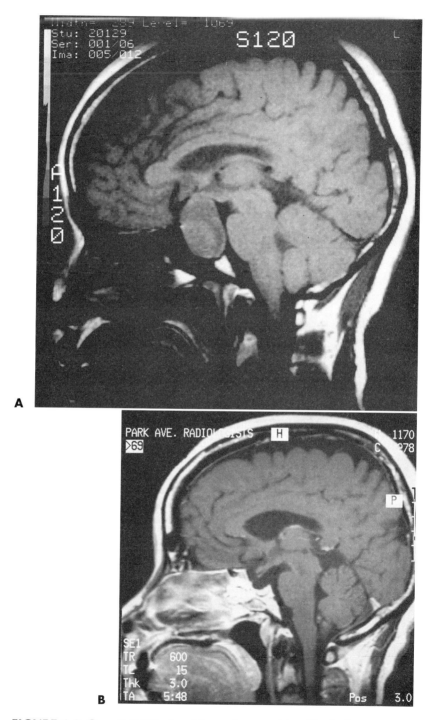

FIGURE 6-8 Case 9: MRI of a chiasmal mass, identified after removal as a pituitary adenoma, **A**, and following removal of the tumor, **B**.

CLINICAL PEARL

Visual field improvements may be seen following tumor removal, after treatment of infections of the retina or brain, and even occasionally in chronic open angle glaucoma.

Summary

In some patients low vision is temporary, and in others it is permanent. Visual field testing plays an important role in determining the etiology and providing information regarding the extent of visual loss. In addition, it can help in following the patient whose vision is changing, and it provides a graphical illustration of the changes that are taking place, allowing the patient to understand the nature of the disorder and the limitations it places on his or her activities. This, in turn, can aid the eye care practitioner in managing treatment and, ultimately, can foster a better relationship between the doctor and low vision patient.

7

Clinical Implications of Color Vision Deficiencies

Michael L. Fischer

Key Terms

Color vision	Farnsworth D-15	Pseudoisochromatic
Acquired defects	Farnsworth-Munsell	plate tests
Color vision testing	100-Hue	PV-16

Why Assess Color Vision at All?

It is probably a fair statement that, although many clinicians may *ask* low vision patients about their color vision, far fewer actually *perform* color vision tests routinely on those patients. There are a number of reasons why this may be so.

First, knowledge of a patient's color vision is not likely to influence patient care and management in most low vision cases. As evidence, consider that some notable texts on low vision care discuss color vision only peripherally. For example, Faye[1] offers one paragraph that briefly mentions the types of color vision defects that may occur in low vision patients and later discusses one test for evaluating children. Mehr and Freid[2] suggest that information about color discrimination can be used to assess central visual function and also prognostically to determine if an individual will be a "successful" low vision patient. They briefly discuss acquired defects and recommend one test for evaluating patients. In both these texts color vision does not play a role in patient *management*. Jose[3] discusses color vision to a slightly greater extent, in terms of testing, rehabilitation, and orientation and mobility; but again, in his volume, it is not a particularly significant factor in low vision care. In other texts (Fonda,[4] Faye and Hood[5]) color vision is not discussed at all. This certainly implies that patients can be managed quite adequately without information about their color discrimination.

Second, most low vision practitioners recognize that psychological and emotional factors play an important role in whether a patient is ready to accept the type of assistance that can be offered at the low vision evaluation. Suppose a patient is having significant difficulty dealing with vision loss but reports no difficulties distinguishing colors. If it is determined that there is a color deficit (even with simple color naming), notifying the patient of this may only exacerbate his or her emotional state. It is questionable if anything positive would be achieved in the long run, especially since most tasks involved in daily living do not depend on a person's color discrimination, and color vision deficiencies, whether acquired or hereditary, cannot be corrected anyway.

So, why bother to test the color vision of the low vision patient? Despite the above discussion, there are two reasons to consider performing color tests on these patients: (1) *Diagnosis*—color test results, in conjunction with other examination findings, can sometimes be a valuable part of a diagnostic profile, when the etiology of a patient's vision loss is uncertain. (2) *Function*—some patients may depend on color discrimination for certain tasks in their daily lives. Knowing which colors are confused may allow the low vision practitioner to counsel the patient (or others working with the patient) on color selection, or on alternate cues or methods of identification, that will help optimize the patient's visual function. The doctor may find color vision testing useful for one or both of these reasons in any particular case. This chapter is intended to present some practical considerations when performing color testing.

Considerations in Color Vision Testing

Whether a test is being done for diagnostic purposes or as part of a functional assessment, it is first necessary to consider the color tests themselves and how they are administered. If the limitations of a particular test are not understood or if the test is performed under improper conditions, the doctor may draw incorrect conclusions. Knowing the right way to perform the test, and what the results mean, will make the information more valuable in patient management.

In the following discussion, it is assumed that the reader has some degree of familiarity with the different types of color vision tests. References are provided for those wishing more in-depth information on both the color tests and the classification of color vision defects.[6,7]

Commercially Available Tests—What They Test

Since the majority of low vision patients who have color defects will have *acquired* color deficiencies secondary to retinal or optic nerve disease, it would be ideal to use a test designed to differentiate among acquired defects. However, in considering the use of color vision tests as diagnostic tools, perhaps the most important point to remember is that most commercially available color vision tests were designed to detect and classify *hereditary* color vision deficiencies. The colors chosen for these tests are very specific (viz., those that fall along the confusion lines of dichromats). Thus, such tests may have limited value with the low vision patient.

CLINICAL PEARL

*Most commercially available color vision tests were designed to detect and classify **hereditary** color vision deficiencies; as such, they may have limited value with the low vision patient.*

Of the tests available, those capable of detecting tritan ("blue-yellow") as well as protan and deutan ("red-green") defects generally will be more useful in patients with ocular disease, since several acquired deficiencies display confusions that more closely resemble tritan-type defects. Many tests are designed to screen out only protan and deutan color deficiencies from the normal population.

Table 7-1 lists some color vision tests currently in use and the types of defects they are designed to detect. Note that, in assembling this table, no judgments have been made as to the validity and reliability of the tests. There are texts available[6,7] that contain detailed summaries of the various tests, along with information and references about validity and reliability studies. Suffice to say, some of the tests have been shown to have greater validity than others, but generally they do what they claim to do.[8-10]

It should be mentioned that arrangement tests, such as the Farnsworth-Munsell 100-Hue Test (FM 100) (see color plate 17), and the Farnsworth Dichotomous Test for Color Blindness—Panel D-15 (D-15) (see color plate 18), tend to be more flexible in terms of their use in disease evaluation because the test design allows the patient to "create" the defect, based on the arrangement of components in the test. As such, patients are not limited to making the color confusions common with hereditary deficiencies but can display whatever types of confusion they may be seeing. (NOTE: A weakness of the 100-Hue Test is that it is too time consuming to be practical for many clinicians to use.) Pseudoisochromatic plate (PIP) tests (see color plate 19) are the more popular form of color vision screening instrument and are used by most practitioners.

TABLE 7-1
Capabilities of Some Color Tests Currently in Use

Test	Distinguishes "red-green" from normals	Distinguishes protans from deutans	Distinguishes "blue-yellow" (tritans) from normals	Quantifies R-G defect to 2 or 3 levels
Pseudoisochromatic Plate Tests				
American Optical Corporation Pseudoisochromatic Plates for Testing Color Perception	Yes			
AO-HRR (Hardy-Rand-Rittler) Plates	Yes	Yes	Yes	Yes (3)
City University Colour Vision Test	Yes	Yes	Yes	
Color Vision Testing Made Easy™	Yes			Yes (2)
Dvorine Color Perception Test Charts*	Yes	Yes		Yes (3)
Farnsworth F2 Tritan Plate	(R-G defect will affect results)		Yes	
Ishihara's Tests for Colour-Blindness†	Yes	Yes		Yes (2)
Standard Pseudoisochromatic Plates for Congenital Color Vision Defects (SPP-C)	Yes	Yes		Yes (3)
Standard Pseudoisochromatic Plates for Acquired Color Vision Defects (SPP-A)	Yes		Yes	
Tokyo Medical College Plate Test	Yes	Yes	Yes	Yes (3)
Arrangement Tests				
Farnsworth Dichotomous Test for Color Blindness (Panel D-15)‡	More severe only	Yes	Yes	(Milder defects will pass)
Farnsworth-Munsell 100-Hue Test	Yes	Yes	Yes	(Score relates to severity)

Compiled from Pokorny et al.,[6] Ichikawa et al.,[11,22] American Optical,[12] Hardy et al.,[13] Farnsworth,[23] Honson et al.,[24] Pinckers et al.,[25] Hyvärinen,[26] and Waggoner.[57]
*A two-card screening version is included as part of the Keystone Visual Skills Test Set.
†Comes in 14, 24, and 38 plate editions, but all have the same capability.
‡Also comes in jumbo and desaturated versions (Plate 18); the children's color test by Hyvärinen uses the same hues as the D-15 and has larger caps.

Unfortunately, however, their value in testing for acquired defects is more limited because the color confusions that can be tested are preselected.

Acuity and Contrast Considerations

Visual acuity and contrast sensitivity are almost always issues with the low vision population, and they may be the most important considerations in testing these patients. The degree to which a patient's acuity is a factor in color vision testing may depend to some extent on the type of test being used. Pseudoisochromatic plate tests involve having the patient identify a figure of one color or set of colors (generally a number, shape, or traceable path) embedded in a background of a different color. Manufacturers of most of these tests[7] suggest that the patient should have better than 20/200 acuity to be able to see the figures. Obviously this could be a limitation to the use of such tests with low vision patients.

A patient who has better than 20/200 acuity may still have difficulty with a PIP test, possibly because there is insufficient contrast between the figure and the ground. Or the patient might have difficulty with the figure-ground task itself. The numbers used in the PIP test are sometimes hard to identify, even for a patient with no vision problems. If figure-ground is believed to be the problem, having the patient trace what is seen with a cotton-tipped applicator may help (testing instructions[11–13] recommend that patients not use their fingers since oil and dirt from the skin can damage the test). Frequently, after tracing the figure, the patient is able to identify it.

Acuity is less important if arrangement tests (D-15, FM 100) are used, since these tests incorporate a matching task rather than identification of a figure. Even the size of the test elements is not extremely limiting in terms of the patient's acuity. For example, it is recommended that the D-15 test be performed at about 50 cm. At this distance the colored caps subtend 1.5°,[6] which is approximately equivalent in size to an 8M letter at the same distance. Therefore, the patient with an acuity reduction of 20/400 should still be able to see the caps and perform the test. Furthermore, the angular subtense of the caps can be increased simply by holding them closer to the eye, making the test somewhat easier for the low vision patient. Obviously a patient could have worse than 20/200 acuity and still attempt to perform this type of task.

Jumbo versions of the D-15 have also been developed for testing low vision patients. One, by Ehrnst and Georgeson (see color plate 18), has caps 30 mm across, which is 2.5 times larger than the standard D-15 test. Others have been used in some studies[14–17] that were up to 8 times larger than the standard test, but these were not commercially available. Some studies[17–21] have reported that test performance by low vision patients improves with larger test elements, in comparison to performance with the standard versions of the D-15, but this finding has not been consistent.

Test Sensitivity

In the performance of color vision testing, it is useful to know not only what types of defects the test can detect (as discussed earlier) but how sensitive the test is. Many times you may draw an inappropriate conclusion about the severity of a patient's color defect because of not being aware of the sensitivity of the test.

For example, a patient might display a classic deutan color deficiency on the D-15 test, but also report no problems seeing colors and be able to name the colors of most objects. From this history the examiner might conclude that the patient has only a mild deficiency, when in fact the patient most likely has a relatively severe deficiency. The D-15 was designed more along the lines of an occupational test, so people who have only mild deficiencies usually pass it with little or no difficulty while people who fail it are usually closer to the "severe" end of the color deficiency continuum. Conversely, PIP tests (e.g., the Ishihara) are generally *very sensitive* for hereditary deficiencies and will detect people who have even the mildest color defect (provided it is one the test picks up).

CLINICAL PEARL

People who fail the D-15 test are usually closer to the "severe" end of the (hereditary) color deficiency continuum.

Some plate tests allow the examiner to more critically assess the severity of a color defect (see Table 7-1). The American Optical–Hardy-Rand-Rittler (AO-HRR) PIP test, for example, has plates that not only help distinguish among protans, deutans, and tritans but also assist in classifying the defect as mild, moderate, or severe. However, be aware that there are other considerations besides test validity (e.g., lighting and test distance, to be discussed) that can influence test results and thus affect the sensitivity and specificity of any particular test.

When performing a color vision evaluation for diagnostic purposes, it is best not to rely on the results of a single test but rather to perform a battery of tests to determine the type and severity of color deficiency. This will provide you with greater information and allow a more accurate assessment of the patient's color perception. Unfortunately, the PIP tests may have limited use in the low vision population for other reasons (reduced acuity and contrast), thus limiting your ability to utilize a test battery.

Lighting

Because the color of an object is based on the wavelengths of light it reflects or transmits, the light source used to illuminate the object can influence its color. Most standard color vision tests (those that do not have their own illumination systems) are hue discrimination tasks and as such have been designed so that saturation (the amount of white in the mixture) and brightness do not influence them. They also have been designed to be used under standard illuminant "C," a bluish light that is intended to mimic northern skylight and has a color temperature of around 6774 K.[6]

If the light source being used for color testing does not provide all wavelengths, it can change the characteristics of the test. For example, many fluorescent lights tend to have peaks of transmission at certain wavelengths and some have broad bands of missing wavelengths. Incandescent bulbs provide too much light in the red end of the spectrum. Using either of these on a PIP test may actually provide the patient with contrast cues (because some of the colors may not be illuminated as brightly) and lead you to either miss a subtle defect or misinterpret the severity of a defect. There are a number of reports in the literature[27-33] addressing the issue of color testing under different light sources and how it changes the characteristics of the test. Richards et al.,[34] evaluating different types of light sources on certain color tests, concluded that some fluorescent sources are adequate for clinical use or screening, but critical evaluation of color vision still necessitates using an appropriate light source.

The light source that is commonly used for critical color vision evaluation is the Macbeth Easel Lamp, which provides source "C" light. But, of course, most clinicians do not have a Macbeth lamp. If the choice of light source is limited to standard incandescent or fluorescent lamps, you will likely get a more valid result using an incandescent source, in conjunction with an appropriate daylight filter (available at photography stores). A daylight filter will raise the color temperature to a more appropriate level. However, for the low vision patient with reduced acuity, using an incorrect illuminant will probably not greatly influence the test results in many cases.

Monocular or Binocular?

Whether testing is done monocularly or binocularly depends, to some extent, on why you are doing it. If it is because you need diagnostic information, remember that most (though not all) hereditary color defects are symmetrical while acquired deficiencies are frequently different between the two eyes. It is therefore essential that color testing always be performed monocularly when done for diagnostic purposes. As with other diagnostic tools, an interocular difference can be a very significant finding. However, if you are performing the test strictly to see how the low vision patient is functioning (in terms of confusing colors or naming colors), it is usually sufficient to perform it binocularly.

Other Considerations

Other factors (e.g., viewing distance, length of presentation of the test elements, the test itself) must be considered in the evaluation of a patient's color vision. Some studies[35,36] have reported that changing parameters like viewing distance and presentation time can change test results in patients with normal visual function. These factors may be important in evaluating low vision patients as well, but for different reasons. Closer test distances make the test elements larger, which may make the test easier for the patient with reduced acuity to perform. Similarly, letting the low vision patient view the test elements for longer periods may allow him to adjust fixation (perhaps finding a better-functioning portion of the retina) and permit improved performance to occur, as sometimes happens during acuity testing. The studies cited did not consider these specific issues.

Instructional sets also can play an important role in the test results, particularly on arrangement tests where the patient's task is to place the caps in order by color. Many times a patient will not understand what this means, and sloppy instructions can result in a totally confusing response, even though the patient actually has no significant color defect. On the D-15, for example, it is often preferable to explain the test to the patient, instruct him or her to find the cap that most closely matches the reference cap, and then wait until this is done. Once the first cap is placed, the instructions are given again ("find the cap that most closely matches the one you have placed in the box"). And, after each cap is placed, the instructions are repeated until you are confident the patient understands the test (perhaps two to four times). This can help eliminate errors in the interpretation of instructions.

There are strengths and weaknesses to almost every available color vision test, but discussing these in detail would require an entire chapter. The point is, if you plan to perform a color test to get diagnostic information, remember that it has its limitations, as does any other diagnostic tool, and the results need to be assessed in the context of the entire clinical picture.

A Word about Filters

It should be no surprise that colored filters have the potential to change a person's color perception. Thomas and Kuyk[37] have reported on the changes in performance on the D-15 test that occur when patients with normal color vision take the test wearing various popular forms of sun wear that absorb in the short-wavelength region, including some absorptive lenses commonly used by low vision practitioners. A few of the filters (Corning CPF 550, NoIR amber 40%) produced no significant change in the D-15 results. One, however (Vuarnets), produced color confusions that looked very much like a tritan ("blue-yellow") defect. As noted earlier, defects following the blue-yellow axis can be indicative of an acquired deficiency.

The point: be aware of the presence of a tint in the patient's spectacle or contact lens prescription. A tint not only can affect test results but, in some cases, may produce or exaggerate color confusions in the patient during everyday activities. Any tinted lens should be removed before testing, and a trial lens correction used if acuity is a consideration for the test.

Finally, a comment about filters to "correct color blindness"—a question you may have been asked at some point. There are no filters that will correct a color deficiency (whatever the cause). Although a filter may give the color-deficient observer clues as to what colors might be present, it does not significantly improve that person's ability to identify colors. The classical story most of us have heard is about the color-deficient observer who fails the Ishihara test and then retakes it using a red filter and sees all the plates. (His color vision is corrected!) Unfortunately, all that has really happened is that he now is identifying the numbers via contrast cues (only the red comes through the red filter, everything else turns essentially gray or black). If you ask him to name the color of an object that he normally has trouble naming while wearing the filter, the odds are he will still name it incorrectly and in fact may have greater difficulty naming it. (I have informally done this with patients using the D-15.) Such a filter has limited use in daily activities.

CLINICAL PEARL

There are no filters that will correct a color deficiency. Filters may give the color-deficient observer other clues to what colors might be present, but they do not significantly improve that person's ability to identify colors.

A colored filter may be used appropriately for the patient with a color deficiency to assist in performing a specific color-discrimination task. With the appropriate filter, and by proper education as to how objects will look through it (e.g., viewed through a red filter, green objects will appear black), you may be able to assist certain individuals in very specific situations. However, it is inappropriate to suggest to them that their color vision can be corrected.

Characteristics of Acquired Color Vision Deficiencies

Comparison of Hereditary and Acquired Defects

Any good text on color vision will contain a thorough discussion of the characteristics of hereditary color vision deficiencies. My intent here is not to discuss this in detail. However, since most low vision patients present with acquired defects secondary to some disease process, you should have a basic understanding of the characteristics of hereditary (congenital) color defects to be able to distinguish them from acquired defects. It is also important to note that changes in color perception resulting from ocular disease occur by a very different mechanism from the one operating in hereditary deficiencies. Congenital defects occur because of the altered characteristics of the cone photopigments themselves, leading to classical types of color confusions. But, remember, you are dealing with an otherwise healthy and normal eye. In

TABLE 7-2
Hereditary versus Acquired Color Vision Deficiencies

Hereditary (congenital)	Acquired
Usually males (X-linked)	Male or female
Usually "red-green" type of defect	Can be "blue-yellow" or "red-green"
Predictable results on color vision tests (classical confusions across different tests)	Unpredictable results (area of loss often not definable)
Repeatable results	Often not repeatable
Usually symmetrical in both eyes	Often asymmetrical in the two eyes
Color defect is stable	Defect may change over time
Name colors of many objects correctly (may name all correctly depending on type and degree of defect)	Incorrectly name some object colors (sometimes reporting sudden difficulty)
Color vision less dependent on target size and illuminance	Color vision very dependent on target size and illuminance
Otherwise normal visual function in most cases	Frequently show other abnormal visual functions (reduced visual acuity, visual field loss, affected contrast sensitivity)

acquired deficiencies (as expected in the low vision population), patients start off with *normal* color vision systems, and changes take place that are likely to affect not only their color perception but other aspects of their visual function as well. Table 7-2 summarizes some of the basic differences between hereditary and acquired deficiencies.

Classifying Acquired Color Vision Defects

Because the characteristics of acquired defects are very different from hereditary ones, it is inappropriate to classify them in the same way. For instance, while a patient may display a defect that looks "sort of deutan" on one particular test, it may not be a consistent finding across a variety of tests, as would occur with hereditary deficiencies. Furthermore, the defect may change as the disease progresses. The terms *protan*, *deutan*, and *tritan* therefore should be reserved for classifying hereditary defects since they imply specific and stable types of color confusions.

Other methods of classifying acquired defects have been reported over the years. Many clinicians are, no doubt, familiar with Köllner's law,[38] which states that lesions of the outer retinal layers give rise to "blue-yellow" types of defects while lesions of the inner retinal layers and optic nerve give rise mainly to "red-green" defects. Whereas this is certainly easy to remember, it tends to be an oversimplification and does not hold true in all instances. A more comprehensive classification for acquired defects was proposed by Verriest,[39] which categorizes most of these defects into three major groups—type I acquired red-green ("sort of protan"), type II acquired red-green ("sort of deutan"), and type III acquired blue-yellow ("sort of tritan"). For interested readers, a thorough discussion of the Verriest system can be found in Pokorny et al.[6]

The points you need to keep in mind when assessing a patient's acquired color deficiency are that (1) the defect may resemble a hereditary loss, but the mechanism is very different; (2) it is quite possible you will not be able to classify an acquired defect because the color confusions appear random (Figs. 7-1 and 7-2); and (3) even if you can

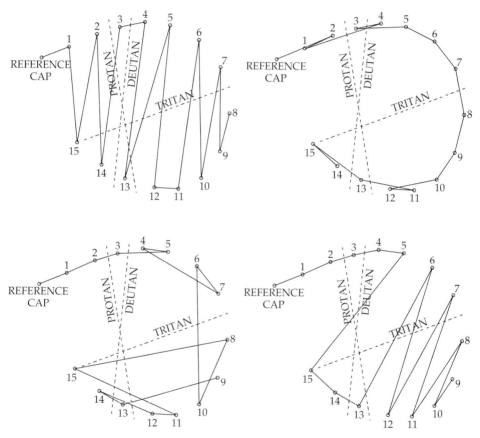

FIGURE 7-1 D-15 results in four separate conditions. **Top left:** A typical outcome for a deuteranope (hereditary defect). Note that the confusions (crossings) follow the deutan axis. **Top right:** A patient with age-related macular degeneration. Changes in the blue-green region (caps 1 to 4) and the purple region (caps 11 to 15) are typical in conditions like age-related macular degeneration and glaucoma and in patients with yellowing of the crystalline lens. **Bottom left:** The result produced by a patient with Leber's optic atrophy. Note that the errors are random and do not follow any axis. **Bottom right:** The results of a patient who matches on the basis of perceived brightness *only*—a patient with achromatopsia (Courtesy Dr. Alan Lewis).

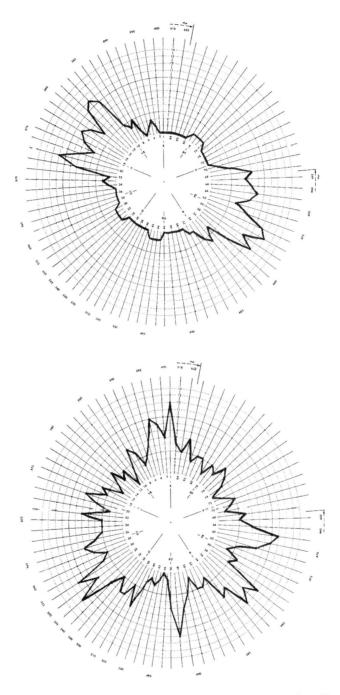

FIGURE 7-2 Examples of Farnsworth-Munsell 100-Hue results. **Top:** A patient with a deutan deficiency. The errors are predominantly in two areas (a bipolar distribution typical of hereditary defects). **Bottom:** A patient with a meningioma. These errors are random around the circle.

classify a defect as "blue-yellow" or "red-green," it may change over time. In other words, for diagnostic purposes, do not put too much weight on the results of a color vision test; also keep the information in the context of an entire diagnostic profile.

Reported Acquired Color Deficiencies

Table 7-3 lists alphabetically some of the conditions that you may likely encounter, with the types of associated color defects ("blue-yellow" or "red-green"). Refer to Table 7-1 to see if the particular test you are using might be better for a particular condition.

It is also common for pharmaceutical agents to produce changes in color perception, either as a possible side effect at normal dosages or secondary to drug toxicity. Many of these changes probably result from damage to the retina (e.g., with chloroquine) or optic nerve (e.g., with ethambutol) that may occur with the agents, and therefore the concomitant color defects reported would seem to make sense.

TABLE 7-3
Common Conditions of the Visual System and Associated Color Defects*

Condition	Frequently Reported Color Confusions
Amblyopia (functional with central fixation)	None (normal)
Cataracts (nuclear yellowing only)	"Blue-yellow"
Central areolar choroidal dystrophy	"Red-green?" (may be normal)
Central serous choroidopathy	"Blue-yellow"
Choroiditis or chorioretinitis	"Blue-yellow" (less often red-green)
Compressive lesions (optic nerve or chiasm)	"Red-green"
Cone dystrophy	"Red-green"
Diabetic retinopathy	"Blue-yellow"
Glaucoma	"Blue-yellow"
Hypertensive retinopathy	"Blue-yellow"
Macular degeneration, age-related	"Blue-yellow"
Macular degeneration (Stargardt's)	"Red-green"
Malignant neoplasms	"Blue-yellow"
Myopic degeneration	"Blue-yellow" (often normal if macula intact)
Ocular hypertension	"Blue-yellow"
Optic atrophy (autosomal dominant)	"Blue-yellow"
Optic atrophy (Leber's)	"Red-green"
Optic neuritis (includes retrobulbar)	"Red-green"
Optic neuropathy (ischemic)	"Blue-yellow"
Papilledema	"Blue-yellow"
Papillitis	"Red-green"
Retinal detachment	"Blue-yellow"
Retinitis pigmentosa	"Blue-yellow", "red-green", achromatopsia, normal
Sickle cell retinopathy	"Blue-yellow"
Vascular occlusion (retinal artery or vein)	"Blue-yellow"

---

*Remember: These are relative tendencies **only**. Defects may not be present at all or may display no clearcut pattern.[6,39,40]

With the tremendous number of drugs now available, it should be no surprise that there are literally hundreds with which color vision disturbances have been reported. Thus it is virtually impossible to detail this information. Table 7-4 combines data from various sources[6,41–43] in an attempt to list some agents that you may encounter in a routine history taking. You may wish to refer to a pharmaceutical or pharmacology reference text for more information on the incidence of color vision disturbances from these and other agents.

Again, it bears repeating: acquired color deficiencies from either diseases or drugs can be quite variable and may or may not resemble

TABLE 7-4

Reported Changes in Color Vision from a Few Common Pharmaceutical Agents

Purpose of Agent	Specific Drugs or Drug Group	Reported Color Defects on Tests	Other Reported Chromatopsias*
Analgesic/Antipyretic	Acetaminophen	—	Yellow vision
	Aspirin (salicylates)	"Red-green" (transient)	Yellow vision, others
	Ibuprofen	"Red-green"	—
Anorexiant	Amphetamines	—	Blue vision
Antibiotic	Chloramphenicol	"Red-green"	Yellow vision
	Erythromycin	"Blue-yellow"	Nonspecific dyschromatopsias
	Nalidixic acid	—	Yellow, blue, or purple vision
	Streptomycin	"Red-green"	Yellow vision
	Sulfonamides	"Red-green"	Yellow or blue vision
	Tetracycline	"Blue-yellow" (transient)	Yellow vision
Anticonvulsant	Phenytoin	—	Colors appear faded
Antidepressant	MAO inhibitors	"Red-green"	Yellow vision
Antimalarial	Chloroquine	"Blue-yellow" (also "red-green")	Yellow vision, others
	Quinine	"Red-green"	Red, green, or yellow vision, others
Antipsychotic	Phenothiazines	"Blue-yellow" (also "red-green")	Yellow or brown vision
Antitubercular	Ethambutol	"Red-green " (may be "blue-yellow")	Nonspecific dyschromatopsias
Cardiovascular	Digitalis glycosides	"Blue-yellow"/ "Red-green"	Yellow vision
	Diuretics	—	Yellow vision
	Quinidine	"Red-green"	Nonspecific dyschromatopsias
Nutrient	Vitamin A	—	Yellow vision
Oral contraceptive	Various	"Blue-yellow" (also "red-green")	Blue vision
Sedative/Hypnotic	Barbiturates	—	Yellow or green vision
	Ethyl alcohol	"Red-green"	Nonspecific dyschromatopsias
	Methyl alcohol†	"Blue-yellow"	—

Compiled from Pokorny et al.,[6] Fraunfelder,[41] Bartlett and Jaanus,[42] and Lyle.[43]
*Example: Yellow vision (xanthopsia) refers to objects having a yellow tinge, etc.
†Methyl alcohol is included here for comparison with ethyl alcohol.

hereditary defects. Tables 7-3 and 7-4 show only the tendencies. They should be used merely as guidelines.

Testing the Low Vision Patient in a Practice Setting

What can you, the private practitioner, accomplish with the color test(s) already in your office? Of course, the answer partly depends on which tests you own. More flexibility in testing for acquired deficiencies will be possible if a test can assess "blue-yellow" confusions in addition to "red-green." And, clearly, a test that is relatively quick and easy to administer is always desirable. Another consideration is *why* you are doing the testing. As discussed at the start of this chapter, you may be performing the test to get information for the patient's diagnostic profile, or for functional reasons (to see which colors the patient confuses in everyday activities).

Testing for diagnostic purposes

If diagnostic information is sought, of the tests more commonly used today the D-15 seems to be one of the best for evaluating the low vision patient. In their respective texts, Mehr and Freid[2] and Jose[3] cite the D-15 as a test of choice. It can detect, and possibly categorize, some acquired color deficiencies with relative speed and simplicity. And, for the low vision patient, the arranging task may be easier to perform than the figure-ground form-recognition tasks utilized with pseudo-isochromatic plate tests.

If using the test to obtain diagnostic information, however, there are certain considerations you should remember.

First, the D-15 is a less sensitive test and therefore can miss subtle defects that might be present early in a condition. (Presumably the low vision patient is not in an early stage of his eye condition, since acuity changes are more likely to occur in more advanced stages.) Adams et al.[44] have suggested that modifying the scoring procedure for the test can increase its sensitivity. In the D-15 manual,[23] Farnsworth defines a "test failure" as one in which two "major" errors are made—with a "major" error resulting from colors across the color circle being placed next to each other. In recording this result, lines would be seen to connect numbers across the circle (e.g., the results for a deuteranope in Figure 7-1). A normal response would be one in which the caps are ordered consecutively, and the plot would be a line around the circle. Because patients with ocular disease often make errors that do not cross the circle (as in Figure 7-1, an ARMD patient), by Farnsworth's criterion they would not fail.

Adams et al.[44] recommend the following modified pass-fail criterion: "Test failure results when a subject makes more than one single-place error or any error greater than single place." By this method, subtle errors are now considered significant. (NOTE: Because factors like understanding instructional sets and patient attention can affect test performance, some degree of *repeatability* is also important in terms of significance of these small errors.)

A second consideration in using the D-15 in ocular disease assessment was touched on earlier: The results frequently cannot be defined as easily as in hereditary deficiencies. Often the errors are only single place in various parts of the color circle or, if "major," do not follow any particular axis (see Fig. 7-1). In either case the area of discrimination loss often cannot be identified. The clinician can, however, be aware of certain trends. For example, patients with conditions that produce a milder loss in blue sensitivity may show single-place errors or errors of just a few places (e.g., putting cap 11 and cap 14 next to each other). These more often will appear in the blue-green and purple regions of the test and may occur in conditions like macular degeneration, diabetic retinopathy, glaucoma, and nuclear sclerosis of the lens. As the loss in blue sensitivity becomes more significant, "major" errors may be produced following the tritan axis on the recording sheet.

In a similar fashion, diseases that can produce color vision losses categorized by Verriest as Type I and Type II red-green defects may demonstrate errors that run in a similar direction to the protan or deutan axis (or somewhere between the two). It is also possible that, as some conditions progress and more damage occurs, errors will be produced along a "scotopic" axis (see Fig. 7-1). This results from the patient's making matches based solely on perceived brightness (the same result as might be produced by a patient with congenital achromatopsia). Unfortunately, many times the errors will merely be random. The point is that although the D-15 (and other standard tests) may allow the *detection* of a problem it is often difficult to *classify* the defect.

CLINICAL PEARL

*Although the D-15, 100-Hue, or other tests may allow the **detection** of an acquired color vision problem, it is often difficult to **classify** the defect.*

Another clinical test that has been designed recently is the *PV-16* quantitative color vision test by Hyvärinen.[26] This test, designed for use with children, utilizes the same hues as the D-15 but has larger-sized caps which subtend 3.8° at 50 cm (more than twice the size of the regular D-15). You have the option of putting a restricting ring on the caps to make them approximately the same size as the D-15 caps. The test can be performed exactly the same way as the D-15, as an "arranging" task, but for the young child who does not understand the concept of putting the caps in order or selecting the cap of the closest color, you may administer the test as a "matching" task (two complete sets of caps are provided for this purpose). Hyvärinen suggests a specific testing procedure when evaluating the young child, and she discusses ways to identify if the child has a color deficiency (the test results are ultimately plotted the same way as in the D-15). Because of the larger cap sizes, this test may also be useful in low vision adult patients.

In discussing arrangement tests, the Farnsworth-Munsell 100-Hue should also be mentioned. Even though most practitioners do not have this test in their offices, referral for the test may be appropriate and feasible for some patients. The FM-100, although more sensitive than the D-15, has similar limitations in terms of classifying defects. Patients with hereditary deficiencies will classically display a bipolar distribution in their errors on the 100-Hue plot, with the location of the poles defining the defect (Figure 7-2 shows the location of the errors for a deutan defect). It is possible for a patient with an acquired deficiency to also demonstrate confusion in specific areas of the color circle, producing "poles" that may look similar to those in a hereditary defect. If this occurs, classification of the defect (according to Verriest) is obviously possible and makes the information more useful in a diagnostic profile. However, as with the D-15, frequently the defect will follow no particular pattern (see Fig. 7-2, meningioma patient), limiting the value of the information. In cases like this, the magnitude of the error (rather than the direction) is often the significant finding. Progression or regression of the disease may be reflected in an increase or decrease in the error score. Again, one problem with the FM-100 is the time it takes to be administered.

What about the tests used by **most** practitioners, the pseudoisochromatic plate (PIP) tests? Many of these do not allow assessment of "blue-yellow" (tritan) defects, which limits their utility (see Table 7-1). Tests like the Ishihara, however, *can* be used to detect losses in color discrimination resulting from "red-green" defects. These tests may be especially useful in assessing unilateral inflammation of the optic nerve, because the patient likely not only has more difficulty identifying the figures with the affected eye, but may also report the decrease in saturation of colors associated with optic neuritis.

If inflammatory optic nerve disease is suggested (either past or present), there are other quick tests you can perform to assess loss of color saturation in the affected eye. One useful technique[45] is to compare the perceived saturation of a red light between the two eyes. The red light can be produced with a transilluminator and the red cap from a pen or an empty bottle of phenylephrine, tropicamide, or some other parasympatholytic agent. Have the patient cover one eye and view the red light with the open eye. Instruct him to quantify the "redness" of the light in terms of some easily understood units (e.g., "Assume this is a dollar's worth of red"). Then do the same thing with the other eye. If the patient reports only a slight difference (only $0.80 or $1.20 worth of red), it is difficult to draw any definitive conclusion. If a significant difference between the eyes is perceived ($0.50 or $2.00 worth of red compared with the fellow eye), the eye with the lesser value most likely has an optic nerve problem. This finding should, of course, be taken in context with the entire diagnostic picture.

It should also be noted here that, in addition to using standard color vision tests (those originally designed for hereditary deficiencies), you have the option of obtaining a test intended to specifically evaluate acquired deficiencies. A number of these tests are commercially available. One example is the desaturated versions of the D-15 test. Two available versions are the Lanthony Desaturated Panel D-15,[46] and the Adams Desaturated D-15[47] (see color plate 18). The desaturation of colors makes the task of placing the caps in order more difficult, resulting in greater sensitivity. Couple this with Adams' modified scoring criterion and the test becomes even more sensitive, so much so that a small percentage of normal subjects will fail it based on this criterion. The desaturated D-15 has been reported[48] to be sensitive to color perception changes in patients with visible pigmentary changes in the macula but no acuity changes. However, it should also be noted that for low vision patients with significant loss of visual function, the color differences on the desaturated versions of the test may be too subtle for them to perform the test or for you to get any meaningful information.

Some plate tests permit testing of tritan defects (see Table 7-1). One that was designed specifically to assess acquired defects is the Standard Pseudoisochromatic Plates for Acquired Color Vision Defects (SPP-A).[49] Mäntyjärvi[50] reported this test to be useful in screening diabetic patients for color vision defects. The ease of administering a plate test is an advantage. It should be noted, though, that Somerfield et al.,[35] studying the effect of changing viewing conditions, found this test to be significantly affected by changes in viewing distance and duration of presentation. Even under viewing conditions specified by the publishers, errors were made by 90% of *normal* observers. Another PIP test, which has desaturated plates, is the Mark II edition of the City University Colour Vision Test. This has also demonstrated certain poorly performing plates. (NOTE: There are other, newer color vision tests[51-55] that have been developed but are not discussed here because they are not commonly used, have not been fully evaluated [because they are so new], or are of only limited value in the low vision population. Interested readers may wish to investigate these tests further.)

Testing for Functional Purposes

If a patient comes into the office with a known diagnosis, the low vision practitioner who does evaluate color-discrimination ability is most likely doing so for functional rather than diagnostic reasons. In this case the goal is to get a practical sense of what kinds of confusions the patient is making as well as try to determine how any color confusions might be affecting the patient's day-to-day activities.

Although standardized color vision tests (e.g., the D-15) may give some information, the results often do not readily lend themselves to prediction of task performance. If a patient reports having difficulty identifying colors in a specific situation, it is more useful to make the evaluation while he or she is performing the actual task in which the color confusions take place. Even with patients who have hereditary color defects, the only way to know for certain that they can or cannot perform a task is to test them *at the task*. This is especially true for persons with hereditary color defects, who learn to name most or all colors properly based on their altered color vision system.

CLINICAL PEARL

The only way to know for certain that a patient can or cannot perform a particular color-discrimination task (either in daily activities or at work) is to test that person at the task.

Color discrimination may be important to the low vision patient in a variety of situations. Identifying colors may be required on the job. A person may have to sort colored items (forms or files) or distinguish colored objects (wires or LED indicators). Colors may be an important part of one's avocation (e.g., painting, embroidery). And a common complaint of many people with low vision is their inability to distinguish colors of clothing. In this situation a simple "test" (obviously) would be to have the individual try to identify some basic colors in the examination room (caps from mydriatic bottles, pictures, your clothing).

A certain degree of color discrimination may also play a role in the patient's health care. Medications or medication bottles may incorporate colors as a method of identification. Diabetics may need to identify or distinguish colors to monitor certain aspects of their status. Most diabetics today use glucometers with a digital readout to monitor their blood glucose, as opposed to the urine tests (rarely used now), which required color identification or matching.[56] However, it is important for many diabetics also to monitor their ketones, and this test still requires a color-matching task with shades of pink and brown (the brightness differences may be sufficient to allow many diabetics to adequately perform this task).

Other aspects of daily living involve identifying colors. As Jose[3] suggests, color cues may be beneficial to a patient in terms of mobility. Traffic lights are just one example. Color also can be effectively used in the presentation of educational materials and is frequently an important learning tool in the younger grades. And it also may be necessary to have the computer user change color selections on the program he or she is using (e.g., letters vs. background) to optimize performance.

Summary

While color vision testing may not be appropriate for every low vision patient, having information about his or her color vision can be valuable in patient management in certain circumstances. It can be useful in establishing the diagnostic profile, helping the doctor arrive at an appropriate diagnosis. Or it may be a significant part of the functional assessment. You should be careful to pursue in the history whether or not color vision plays a role in the patient's daily lifestyle. If it does, then some type of color vision evaluation should be performed to better manage and counsel the patient.

It is unfortunate that color vision defects cannot be corrected; thus you are limited in the type of assistance that can be offered. There still may be some advice you can extend the patient, however. A colored filter may be of benefit in very specific situations by highlighting a particular color. Sometimes better lighting can improve perception of certain colors. Advice on optimal color selections, or more precisely, on which color combinations to *avoid* (e.g., on a computer screen) may be beneficial to the patient. Ultimately for some, alternate methods of identification of objects (shape, size, labeling) may be the best advice you are able to offer. You never know what may be around the corner, however. Color vision testing has already started making its way into the computer age, as evidenced by the computer-based ColorTest from TwoDocs.[55] With the advances in real time computer imaging that are currently being developed, it may be possible soon to generate a color-enhanced image that provides the color-deficient observer with needed chromatic information to make previously difficult color discriminations easier.

Acknowledgments

Much of the material included in this chapter originally appeared as part of the *Problems in Optometry* series, published by J.B. Lippincott. The figures, the tables (with some modifications), and certain segments of the text came from a chapter by me ("Clinical Color Vision Testing as a Diagnostic Tool," in *Modern Diagnostic Technologies* [vol 3, no. 1 of the series], edited by Paul Abplanalp. I would like to thank Diane Schiumo of the Media Center, State University of New York, College of Optometry, who took the original photographs for plates 18 and 19.

References

1. Faye E: *Clinical low vision*, ed 2, Boston, 1984, Little, Brown.
2. Mehr E, Freid A: *Low vision care*, Chicago, 1975, Professional Press.
3. Jose R (ed): *Understanding low vision*, New York, 1983, American Foundation for the Blind.

4. Fonda G: *Management of the patient with subnormal vision*, St Louis, 1965, Mosby.

5. Faye E, Hood C: *Low vision*, Springfield Ill, 1975, Charles C Thomas.

6. Pokorny J, Smith VC, Verriest G, Pinckers AJ (eds): *Congenital and acquired color vision deficiencies*, New York, 1979, Grune & Stratton.

7. National Research Council, Committee on vision: *Procedures for testing color vision: report of working group 41*, Washington DC, 1981, National Academy Press.

8. Haskett MK, Hovis JK: Comparison of standard pseudoisochromatic plates to the Ishihara Color Vision Test, *Am J Optom Physiol Opt* 64:211-216, 1987.

9. Honson VJ, Dain SJ: Performance of the Standard Pseudoisochromatic Plate Test, *Am J Optom Physiol Opt* 65:561-570, 1988.

10. Adams AJ, Bailey JE, Harwood LW: Color vision screening: a comparison of the AO–H-R-R and Farnsworth F2 tests, *Am J Optom Physiol Opt* 61:1-9, 1984.

11. Ichikawa H, Hukami K, Tanabe SH, Kawakami G: *Standard pseudoisochromatic plates*, New York, 1978, Igaku-Shoin.

12. American Optical Corporation: *Pseudo-isochromatic plates for testing color vision*, Philadelphia, 1965, Beck Engraving.

13. Hardy LH, Rand G, Rittler MC: *AO–H-R-R pseudo-isochromatic plates*, New York, 1957, American Optical.

14. Breton M, Tansley B: Improved color test results with large-field viewing in dichromats, *Arch Ophthalmol* 103:1490-1495, 1985.

15. Steward J, Cole B: The effect of object size on the performance of colour ordering and discrimination tasks. In Drum B, Verriest G (eds): *Colour Vision Deficiencies IX*, (vol. 52), Dordrecht, 1989:79-88, Kluwer Academic Publishers.

16. Motohashi T, Ohta Y, Hanbusa A, Shiraishi H: Comparative study between test results of 8-degree large field anomaloscope and large size D15 test on dichromats. In Drum B, Verriest G (eds): *Colour Vision Deficiencies IX*, (vol. 52), Dordrecht, 1989:543-554, Kluwer Academic Publishers.

17. Knoblauch K, Fischer M, Robillard N, et al.: The effect of test element size on performance of the D-15 in age-related maculopathy and congenital color deficiency. In Drum B, Moreland JD, Serra A (eds): *Colour Vision Deficiencies IX*, (vol 54), *Documenta Ophthalmologica Proceedings Series*, Dordrecht, 1991, Kluwer Academic Publishers.

18. Bailey I, Maino J, Adams A: Color vision testing in low vision patients, *Am J Optom Physiol Opt* 59:40P, 1982.

19. Gresset J, Bolduc M: Comparison of quantitative scores between standard panel D-15 and enlarged panel D-15 in low vision patients, *Am J Optom Physiol Opt* 64:67P, 1987.

20. Sloane M, Kuyk T, Owsley C, et al.: The effects of relative size magnification of Farnsworth D-15 color chips on color vision assessment in low vision patients. In Noninvasive assessment of the visual system, *Techn Dig Ser* 7:140-143, 1989.

21. Knoblauch K, Robillard N, Fischer M, Faye E: Test element size and performance of low vision observers with the panel D-15, *Am J Optom Physiol Opt* 64:60P, 1987.

22. Ichikawa K, Ichikawa H, Tanabe S: Detection of acquired color vision deficiencies by standard pseudoisochromatic plates, part 2. In Verriest G. (ed): *Colour Vision Deficiencies VIII*, (vol 46), The Hague 1987:133-140.

23. Farnsworth D: *The Farnsworth Dichotomous Test for Color Blindness—Panel D-15*, New York, 1947, Psychological Corporation.

24. Honson VJ, Dain SJ: Analysis of the Mark II edition of the City University Colour Vision Test, *Am J Optom Physiol Opt* 64:277-283, 1987.

25. Pinckers A, Nabbe B, Vossen H: Standard pseudoisochromatic plates, part 2, *Ophthalmologica* 190:118-124, 1985.

26. Hyvärinen L: *A large size quantitative color vision test*. Descriptive literature from Precision Vision, Villa Park Ill, 1994.

27. Reed JD: The effect of illumination on changing the stimuli in pseudoisochromatic plates, *J Opt Soc Am* 34:350, 1944.

28. Hardy LH, Rand G, Rittler MC: The effect of quality of illumination on the results of the Ishihara test, *J Opt Soc Am* 36:86-94, 1946.

29. Volk D, Fry GA: Effect of quality of illumination and distance of observation upon performance in the Ishihara test, *Am J Optom Arch Am Acad Optom* 24:99-102, 1947.

30. Farnsworth D, Reed JD, Shilling CW: The effect of certain illuminants on scores made on pseudoisochromatic plate tests, *U.S. Naval medical research, color vision report no 4*, pp 1-9, 1948.

31. Schmidt I: Effect of illumination in testing color vision with pseudoisochromatic plates, *J Opt Soc Am* 42:951-955, 1952.

32. Katavisto M: Pseudo-isochromatic plates and artificial light, *Acta Ophthalmol* 39:377-390, 1961.

33. Higgins K, Moskowitz-Cook A, Knoblauch K: Color vision testing: an alternative "source" of illuminant C, *Mod Probl Ophthalmol* 19:113-21, 1978.

34. Richards OW, Tack TO, Thome C: Fluorescent lights for color vision testing, *Am J Optom Arch Am Acad Optom* 48:747-753, 1971.

35. Somerfield MR, Long GM, Tuck JP, Gillard ET: Effects of viewing conditions on standard measures of acquired and congenital color defects, *Optom Vis Sci* 66:29-33, 1989.

36. Long GM, Lyman BJ, Tuck JP: Distance, duration, and blur effects on the perception of pseudoisochromatic stimuli, *Ophthalmic Physiol Opt* 5:185-194, 1985.

37. Thomas SR, Kuyk T: D-15 performance with short wavelength absorbing filters in normals, *Am J Optom Physiol Opt* 65:697-702, 1988.

38. Köllner H: *Die Storungen des Farbensinnes. Ihre klinische bedeutung und ihre diagnose*, Berlin, 1912, Karger.

39. Verriest G: Further studies on acquired deficiency of color discrimination, *J Opt Soc Am* 53:185-195, 1963.

40. Adams AJ: Chromatic and luminosity processing in retinal disease, *Am J Optom Physiol Opt* 59:954-960, 1982.

41. Fraunfelder FT: *Drug-induced ocular side effects and drug interactions*, Philadelphia, 1982, Lea & Febiger.

42. Jaanus SD, Bartlett JD: Adverse ocular effects of systemic drug therapy. In Bartlett JD, Jaanus SD (eds): *Clinical ocular pharmacology*, Boston, 1984, Butterworths, pp 917-939.

43. Lyle WM: Drug groups potentially able to alter color vision, *Optom Weekly* 67:859-862, 1976.

44. Adams AJ, Rodic R, Husted R, Stamper RL: Spectral sensitivity and color discrimination changes in glaucoma and glaucoma-suspect patients, *Invest Ophthalmol Vis Sci* 23:516-524, 1982.

45. Glaser JS (ed): *Neuroophthalmology*, ed 2, Philadelphia, 1990 JB Lippincott.

46. Lanthony P: The Desaturated Panel D-15, *Doc Ophthalmol* 46:185-189, 1978.

47. Adams AJ, Rodic R: Use of desaturated and saturated versions of the D-15 test in glaucoma and glaucoma-suspect patients. In Verriest G (ed): *Doc Ophthalmol Proc Ser* 33:419-423, 1982.

48. Collins MJ: Pre-age related maculopathy and the Desaturated D-15 Color Vision Test, *Clin Exp Optom* 69:223-227, 1986.

49. Ichikawa H, Hukami K, Tanabe SH: *Standard pseudoisochromatic plates, part 2, For acquired color vision defects*, New York, 1978, Igaku-Shoin.

50. Mäntyjärvi M: Screening of colour vision defects in diabetic patients, *Acta Ophthalmol* 65:178-184, 1987.

51. Adams AJ, Schefrin B, Huie K: New clinical color threshold test for eye disease, *Am J Optom Physiol Opt* 64:29-37, 1987.

52. Estèvez O, Spekriejse H, Van Dalen JTW, Verduyn Lunel HFE: The OSCAR Color Vision Test: theory and evaluation (Objective Screening of Color Anomalies and Reductions), *Am J Optom Physiol Opt* 60:892-901, 1983.

53. Massof RW, Severns ML: The Anomaloscope Plate Test: A new color vision test for screening congenital red-green color vision deficiencies. In Drum B, Verriest G (eds): *Colour Vision Deficiencies IX*, (vol. 52), Dordrecht, 1989:539-541, Kluwer Academic Publishers.

54. Pease P, Allen J: A new test for screening color vision: concurrent validity and utility, *Am J Optom Physiol Opt* 65:729-738, 1988.

55. TwoDocs Inc: ColorTest (computerized color vision test), New Orleans, 1989.

56. Smith V, Burns S, Pokorny J: Colorimetric evaluation of urine-sugar tests used by diabetic patients. In Verriest G (ed): *Doc Ophthalmol Proc Ser* 33:345-354, 1982.

57. Waggoner, TL: *Color Vision Testing Made Easy,* First edition Anaheim, 1994, Home Vision Care (manufacturer).

8

Effective Color Contrast and Low Vision

Aries Arditi
Kenneth Knoblauch

Key Terms

Contrast	Saturation	Color deficit
Chroma	Brightness	Reflectance
Hue	Luminance	Wavelength
Lightness		

Since people can perform most critical pattern processing tasks of everyday life (e.g., reading or driving) even in the absence of hue discrimination capability, chromatic attributes of visual stimuli are generally thought to be of secondary importance in form vision. However, defects and anomalies of color vision that are acquired with eye diseases and produce low vision can affect luminosity and hence effective contrast of most colored visual stimuli. The partially sighted individual whose pattern processing capabilities are already challenged by a high degree of optical and/or neural image degradation often cannot afford additional losses in effective contrast arising from color deficits acquired with ocular disease. In addition, color, especially in graphic displays, often codes information or conveys esthetic features that are important elements of the presentation to the user.

How can colors for information displays be chosen for high discriminability and legibility for individuals with low vision, while still allowing flexibility in color choices? Guidance on this question in the literature is vague, being confined to the mention of color as a cue to enhance visibility of critical environmental features, or to the plea for use of strong color contrasts in designing for partial-sight.[1-3] There has been one recent attempt to provide some guidance in the use of color,[4] but it is neither comprehensive nor easy to generalize.

There are valid reasons for the paucity of specific information guiding the use of color in low vision: color vision deficits vary greatly among eye disorders and individuals. This heterogeneity extends to color appearances, and more important, to discriminability; that is, colors that contrast optimally for one individual may actually be indiscriminable to another. Thus it is not possible to derive a single set of guidelines that are maximally effective for the entire partially sighted population.

Rather than attempt to specify *maximal* effectiveness for each individual, the approach we take here derives, from the most prevalent functional characteristics of color vision loss in low vision, a set of three rules to guide color choices that ought to lead to more effective color choices for the vast majority of partially sighted people. These rules also yield effective contrasts for people with congenital color defects as well, and do not result in less effective contrasts for people with normal color vision.

Hue, Lightness, and Chroma (Saturation)

To understand how to make color contrasts that are effective for everyone, a few basic definitions will be useful. In particular, we need to characterize colors by their three most important perceptual attributes: *hue, lightness,* and *saturation* (see color plate 20).

Hue is the attribute by which colors are categorized with terms like blue, green, yellow, red, and purple. Newton first noted that people with normal color vision report that, when ordered in terms of similarity to one another, hues fall naturally into a closed figure like a circle (see color plate 22).

Lightness (or brightness) is the attribute that corresponds to how much light *appears* to be reflected (or emitted) from a surface relative to that from nearby surfaces. It is the most important attribute in effective contrast between two colors. Notice that different terminology is conventional depending on whether we are referring to the color of surfaces such as walls, whose perceived intensity depends more on the *proportion* of light reflected (or reflectance) rather than on the absolute amount of light coming from the surface, or the color of illuminants such as lamps or the moon, which are seen as sources of light. With the former, we refer to *lightness*; with the latter, *brightness*. Throughout this chapter we refer mostly to lightness, but our rules apply to brightness as well. Another way to think about lightness is as the gray value that appears most similar to the color. Thus pastel colors, which appear to be close to light gray or white, generally have high lightness.

Although it is commonly believed that optical devices such as photographic exposure meters can be used to compute the lightness (or brightness) of a color, they in fact give results that agree only with those of an average observer. The values they register often do not match the observations of many people, especially partially sighted people with acquired deficits and some people with congenital color deficits. Thus one cannot simply measure lightness or brightness (or any other perceptual attribute, for that matter), with an optical device.

Chroma (also called *saturation*) refers to chromatic intensity—the degree to which a surface color differs from an achromatic surface of the same lightness. It is the attribute of color intensity in the sense of its perceptual difference from a white, black, or gray, of equal lightness. Slate blue is an example of a desaturated color, because it is similar to gray. A deep blue of equal lightness to the slate blue would be more saturated.

Because hue, lightness, and saturation can all be abstracted from a stimulus by an observer independently of one another, it is possible to represent perceived color as a solid in three-dimensional space. Illustrated in color plate 20, a **color solid** helps to visualize the three perceptual attributes of color enumerated above. Although the color solid depicted in the figure is highly schematized and is not intended to represent the perceptual color space of any real observer, it has three features worth noting. First, the greatest perceptual distances between colors can be realized by separation on the lightness axis; that is, highest effective contrasts can be achieved by manipulating apparent light intensities. This can be accomplished most directly through changes in actual intensities (luminances or reflectances). Second, the solid is widest in the middle range of lightnesses, reflecting the fact that colors at the lightness extremes have restricted ranges of chroma, and that colors with the highest chroma are found only in the midrange of lightnesses. Thus one can generally increase the apparent intensity of a highly saturated surface or light source only at the expense of its chroma. Finally, hues also tend to be more similar to one another at the lightness extremes.

Color Defects Associated with Low Vision

Most color vision deficits that occur with serious ocular disease are usefully described in terms of the following functional losses.

Luminosity losses. Ocular disorders (and typical aging) often result in a loss of transparency of the ocular media, reducing the amount of light reaching the retina. Such losses are generally greater for short rather than long wavelengths of light. Violet, blue, and blue-green surfaces, which tend to reflect shorter wavelengths, often appear darker to individuals with losses in ocular transparency. Such losses in lightness are often termed luminosity losses. Similarly, certain other eye disorders (cone-rod dystrophies, protan defects, and some forms of achromatopsia) result in loss of luminosity of long wavelength light. For individuals with these types of disorders, surfaces and lights with hues near the red end of the hue scale appear darker.

CLINICAL PEARL

Violet, blue, and blue-green surfaces, which tend to reflect shorter wavelengths, often appear darker to individuals with losses in ocular transparency.

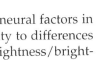

Luminance contrast sensitivity. Many optical and neural factors in eye diseases may contribute to a loss of sensitivity to differences in light intensity. Since apparent light intensity (lightness/brightness) is strongly affected by actual light intensity (luminance), reductions in sensitivity to luminance contrast are also associated with reductions in lightness and brightness contrast.*

CLINICAL PEARL

Because apparent light intensity (lightness/brightness) is strongly affected by actual light intensity (luminance), reductions in the sensitivity to luminance contrast are associated with reductions in the sensitivity to contrast between lightness and brightness.

Chroma discrimination. In many visual disorders, surfaces and lights that are matched in lightness and hue become less discriminable, particularly those that lie close to the achromatic (lightness) axis of the color solid, such as the pastel colors. This is often due to a reduction in the amount of light that reaches the retina

---

*However, since luminance is itself defined in terms of the efficiency of each wavelength to evoke a visual response in a standard normally sighted observer, wavelength-dependent reductions in luminance contrast sensitivity in an individual with a color defect are almost always associated with effects on hue and chroma contrast as well.

because of ocular disease. Chroma discrimination can also be reduced for particular pairs of hues in both congenital and acquired color vision deficits.

CLINICAL PEARL

In many visual disorders, surfaces and lights that are matched in lightness and hue become less discriminable, particularly when they lie close to the achromatic (lightness) axis of the color solid (e.g., pastel-colored objects).

Wavelength discrimination. Color deficits associated with visual impairment also affect the ability to distinguish nearby wavelengths of monochromatic light. Because wavelength is such an important factor in hue, such losses also produce deficits in discriminating adjacent regions of the hue scale.

CLINICAL PEARL

Color deficits associated with visual impairment also affect the ability to distinguish nearby wavelengths of monochromatic light. Because wavelength is such an important factor in hue, such losses produce deficits in discriminating adjacent regions of the hue scale as well.

Three Rules for Obtaining Effective Color Contrast

Given these types of functional losses, a set of three qualitative recommendations is derived for choosing pairs of colors that, if followed, would minimize the likelihood of using color contrasts that are indiscriminable for individuals with low vision. The guidelines are designed to result in choices of color contrasts for which the residual luminance contrast will be good even when an individual has lost the ability to discriminate the chromatic component in the pair. These recommendations are addressed to anyone who wishes to increase the visual accessibility, discriminability, and/or legibility of environments, displays, or colored print materials to patients with low vision. Because of the diversity of color deficits associated with low vision and the fact that we have exploited a statistical association between hue and wavelength composition of lights and ignored adaptation and induction effects, these rules can be incorrect in some instances. However, the rules will be valid for most low vision patients, viewing most colored stimuli under neutral adaptation and illuminating conditions.

1. **Increase lightness differences between foreground and background colors, and avoid using colors of similar lightness against one another, even if they differ in chroma or hue (see color plate 21).** Although the designer cannot be confident that the lightnesses and lightness differences he or she perceives will correspond to the lightnesses and differences perceived by people with color deficits, he or she can generally assume that additional contrast between colors of different lightness will be required for the individual with color deficits. Thus use of lighter light colors and darker dark colors than typically used will increase visual accessibility to all.

CLINICAL PEARL

Increase the lightness differences between foreground and background colors. Also avoid using colors of similar lightness against one another, even if they differ in chroma or hue.

2. **Choose dark colors with hues chosen from the bottom half of the hue circle shown in color plate 22 against light colors from the top half of the circle, and avoid contrasting light colors from colors on the bottom half against light colors on the top half.** Most people with partial sight and/or congenital color deficiency tend to suffer losses in visual efficiency for colors shown in the bottom of this circle; this guideline helps to minimize the deleterious effects of such losses on effective contrast.

CLINICAL PEARL

Choose dark colors, with hues from the bottom half of the hue circle, to accompany light colors, with hues from the top half. Also avoid contrasting light colors from the bottom half against light ones from the top half.

3. **Avoid contrasting hues from adjacent parts of the hue circle (see color plate 23), especially if the colors do not contrast sharply in lightness.** Color deficiencies associated with partial sight (as well as congenital) make colors of similar hue more difficult to discriminate than they are in normal vision.

CLINICAL PEARL

Avoid contrasting hues from adjacent part of the hue circle, especially if they do not differ significantly in lightness.

TABLE 8-1
Color Contrast

Colors	Rule(s)
Good	
Any light color against black	1
Any dark color against white	1
Light yellow against dark blue	2
Dark red against light green	2
Poor	
Dark green against light red	2
Yellow against white or light gray	1
Turquoise against green	3
Lavender against pink	1, 3

Examples

In Table 8-1 above, a few examples are given of good and poor color contrast, as well as the rule(s) applied to classify them as good or poor.

Conclusion

Although the diversity of color deficits in low vision and congenital color deficiency, as well as the diversity of illuminating and adaptation conditions, makes identification of highly specific recommendations very difficult, there are three simple rules that can be applied that are likely to increase effective color contrast in low vision and congenital color deficiency, without decreasing effective contrasts in normal vision. It is hoped that these simple rules will be of value to all who wish their displays to be accessible to individuals with acquired and congenital color deficits.

References

1. Duncan J, Gish C, Mulholland ME, and Townsend A: Environmental modifications for the visually impaired: A handbook. *J Vis Impair Blindness*, 442-455, 1977.
2. Hood CM and Faye EF: Evaluating the living situation. *The Aging Eye and Low Vision.* Lighthouse National Center for Vision and Aging, The Lighthouse Inc., New York, 1992, pp. 46-54.
3. Tideiksaar R: Avoiding falls. *The Aging Eye and Low Vision.* Lighthouse National Center for Vision and Aging, The Lighthouse Inc., New York, 1992, pp. 55-60.
4. Gelhaus MM and Olson MR: Using color and contrast to modify the educational environment of visually impaired students with multiple disabilities. *J Vis Impair Blindness* 19-20, 1993.

9

Electrodiagnosis in Evaluating and Managing the Low Vision Patient

Jerome Sherman
Sherry J. Bass

Key Terms

Visual evoked potential	Retinal degeneration	Optic nerve disease
Electroretinography	Demyelinating disease	Rod monochromatism
Electrooculography	Macular disease	Night blindness

As a low vision practitioner, you are likely to find that on several occasions a patient will present with a history of poor vision and, after your evaluation is complete, you are unable to identify the etiology of the problem. Although there may be associated findings, the cause of the reduced vision sometimes remains a mystery.

Enter the realm of electrodiagnostic testing. Electrodiagnosis is a field in which specific tests are used to assess the function of the retina and optic nerve—tests that do not require any subjective responses and that provide valuable additional information to enable you to determine the etiology. Both you and the patient need to know why the patient's vision is poor. This information is important in determining a prognosis and deciding if other family members are likely to be affected.

CLINICAL PEARL

Electrodiagnosis is a field in which specific tests are used to assess the function of the retina and optic nerve—tests that do not require any subjective responses and that provide valuable additional information to enable you to determine the etiology.

Electrodiagnostic testing is not only objective, it can also be very sensitive to early functional changes in the visual system that precede the manifestations of patient symptoms and clinical signs. In addition, it is valuable in monitoring the progression of disease. A recent clinical trial[1] has shown that vitamin A palmitate can slow the progression of retinitis pigmentosa while vitamin E may be detrimental. Retinitis pigmentosa and all the variants of this disease are the major disease group in which electrodiagnostic testing (specifically the ERG) is extremely valuable in monitoring the progression of disease.

CLINICAL PEARL

Electrodiagnostic testing is not only objective, it can also be very sensitive to early functional changes in the visual system that precede the manifestations of patient symptoms and clinical signs.

The value of early diagnosis using electrodiagnostic testing is manifest when we consider that as the result of recent clinical trials there is, for the first time, an available treatment that has the potential to alter the course of multiple sclerosis, a demyelinating disease that can lead to visual and other disabilities. The drug beta-interferon has been shown[2] to result in 20% fewer MRI-diagnosed brain lesions than in a placebo control group. Optic neuritis, a common finding with demyelinating disease, is the most frequent affliction in which electrodiagnostic testing (specifically the VEP) is most helpful in diagnosis.

CLINICAL PEARL

The value of early diagnosis using electrodiagnostic testing is manifest when we consider that as the result of recent clinical trials there is, for the first time, an available treatment that has the potential to alter the course of multiple sclerosis, a demyelinating disease that can lead to visual and other disabilities.

Now that treatment is available for select visually debilitating conditions, early diagnosis is even more essential. When combined with timely therapeutic intervention, it is in the patient's best interest, and it soon will become the standard of care. Treatment of many of these conditions not only includes pharmaceutical interventions but may also necessitate prescribing specialty lenses. For example, if the results of an electroretinogram enable you to diagnose rod monochromatism, red-tinted spectacles or contact lenses are likely to greatly improve visual function.[3]

Although electrodiagnostic testing has been commercially available for almost 2 decades, it is still an underutilized service, and many low vision patients continue through life never knowing why they cannot see well. Recently, newer systems have been introduced that are more compact, more portable, easier to use, and less costly than their predecessors (Fig. 9-1). They have finally made in-office electrodiagnostic testing a reality.

CLINICAL PEARL

Although electrodiagnostic testing has been commercially available for almost 2 decades, it is still an underutilized service and many low vision patients continue through life never knowing why they cannot see well.

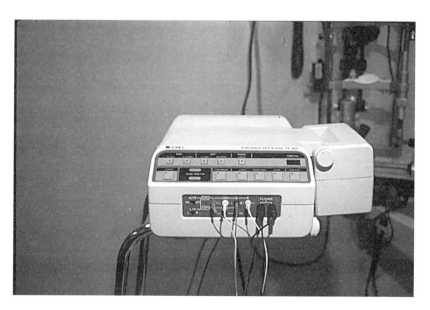

FIGURE 9-1 Electrodiagnostic systems today are easier to use, more portable, and less expensive than their predecessors. (Courtesy Tomey Inc.)

The Visual Evoked Potential

The visual evoked potential (VEP) is an objective test of visual function that can be monitored at the level of the occipital cortex. The electrical activity of the brain, recorded by scalp electrodes, is what constitutes an evoked potential, and when the patient views a visual stimulus the electrical response from the occipital cortex is measured and recorded. Because the response is evoked by a visual stimulus, it is called an **evoked** potential. Compared to other brain activity, the electrical activity evoked by visual stimuli is extremely small. Thus systems to record a VEP must include amplifiers and signal averagers to enlarge the response and minimize background noise so the response can be recorded. The patient does not speak a word and his ability to see can be both qualitatively and quantitatively determined with ease.

CLINICAL PEARL

The patient does not speak a word, and his ability to see can be both qualitatively and quantitatively determined with ease.

There are a multitude of applications for VEP testing—the assessment of refractive error, visual acuity, binocular function, accommodation, and stereopsis, the prognostic determination of amblyopia, and the detection of retinal (macular) and optic nerve dysfunction in the absence of observable pathology or visual symptoms. The objective nature of the VEP makes it an ideal test to perform when evaluating infants and young children, mentally handicapped patients, and patients with psychogenic problems (e.g., hysteria and malingering). Other applications include the presurgical estimate of postsurgical visual function in a patient with media opacities, objective visual field measurements, the assessment of optic nerve damage in glaucoma and orbital disease, objective color vision analysis, the investigation of migraine headaches, the early detection of poisoning, and optic pathway misrouting in albinism, and the objective determination of neurological development. Within the scope of this chapter, however, we will consider only applications in which the patient presents with uncorrectable reduced vision.

Principles and Concepts of VEP Testing

The theoretical aspects and technical considerations of VEP testing are greatly minimized within the context of this chapter, and the reader is referred to other excellent comprehensive sources.[4] The VEP is a cortical response originating primarily from the central retinal cones. This is because the central 5° of the retina comprising the macula project onto about half the occipital cortex. Thus a disproportionately large cortical area corresponds to a small retinal area, since there is an approximately one-to-one relationship between the central retinal cones and the corresponding bipolar and ganglion cells. In addition, the projection of the macula is onto the posterior occipital cortex and is therefore close to the recording electrode. Consequently, the VEP reflects both macular and macular-pathway function.

CLINICAL PEARL

The VEP reflects macular and macular-pathway function.

To perform VEP testing requires the appropriate placement of electrodes, which are usually metal disks or cups connected to a lead wire, that transmit electrical impulses into the computer. The electrodes are attached generally to both earlobes and to the scalp at a point 2.5 cm above the inion (Fig. 9-2). Once they are in place, the patient is directed to look at the visual stimulus, which may be either (a) a screen with a checkerboard pattern of varying sizes in which the checks or squares

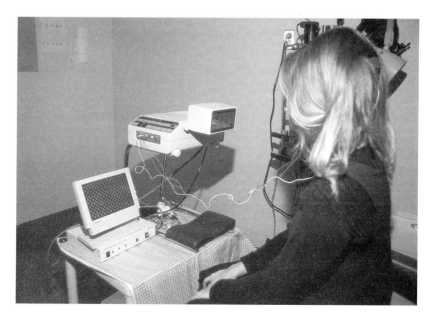

FIGURE 9-2 To set up a patient for a VEP, place the recording electrode 2.5 cm above the inion, the bony protuberance on the back of the head. Then place two other electrodes, a reference and a ground, one on each earlobe. The patient then views the stimulus, in this case a pattern-reversed checkerboard.

change or reverse from dark to light at a specific rate or (b) a bright flashing unpatterned light. The patient is directed to look at the stimulus for about a minute. If a patterned stimulus is being used, the patient must wear his best correction for a 1-meter testing distance and the pupils should not be dilated. To get a "clean" VEP, all noise must be filtered out. Therefore responses will be averaged for this period and the result will appear on the screen or a printout depending on the system being used. Responses can also be affected by other sources of potentials (e.g., neck muscle activity, eye movements, the heartbeat), although these artifacts are usually eliminated by sophisticated software built into the instrument.

The resulting VEP can be either transient or steady-state depending upon the rate at which the checkerboard pattern is reversing. At a slow reversal rate a transient response is generated, which is an individual response to a distinct stimulus. At a faster reversal rate a steady-state response is generated, which is an overlap of responses evoked by a sufficiently high repetition rate. The reversal rate used depends upon the information needed from the test for a specific patient. Figure 9-3, *A*, is

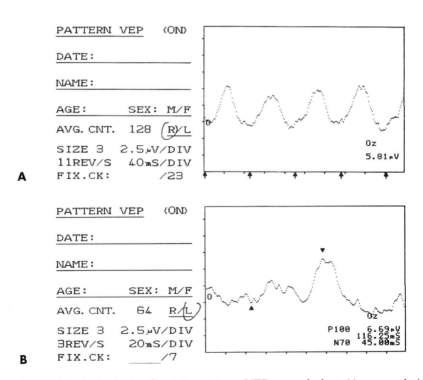

FIGURE 9-3 **A**, A steady-state pattern VEP recorded at 11 reversals/ second. **B**, A transient pattern VEP recorded at a slower rate of 3 reversals/second. Amplitudes and implicit times with the Tomey system are automatically calculated and printed out.

a steady-state VEP that has resulted from the pattern reversal of individual small checks in a large checkerboard. The pattern reversal rate is 3.75 Hz or 7.5 reversals/second (1 Hz = 2 reversals per second). The major responses are a series of sine waves occurring 7.5 times/second. Figure 9-3, *B*, is a transient VEP, which in this case is generated to a slow reversal rate of 1.88 reversals/second. The responses are analyzed for amplitude and latency or implicit time. Amplitudes are measured in microvolts, and latencies in fractions of a second (milliseconds). The expected VEP from a normal eye varies with the size of the pattern or check. A typical pattern stimulus consists of 7, 14, 28, and 56 minute-of-arc checks (i.e., the check size subtending an angle of 7, 14, 28, or 56 minutes of arc at a testing distance of 1 meter). If a normal VEP is recorded to all check sizes presented including the smallest 7 minute-of-arc checks, then the patient is capable of 20/15 to 20/30 visual acuity despite what he may or may not say. (A normal pattern VEP to these check sizes is depicted in Figure 9-4.) On the other hand, if a patient has 20/20 vision and the VEPs are flat to all check sizes, this individual may in fact have a potentially serious problem. Examples are discussed later, under Cases. Typically, though not always, the largest VEP is expected to be in response to the 14 minute-of-arc checks, because this size comes closest to the ganglion cell receptor field size (about 15 minutes of arc).

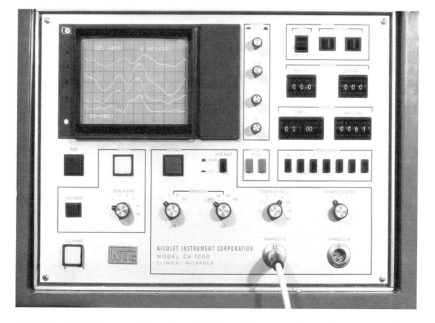

FIGURE 9-4 A normal pattern VEP to checks of varying sizes—from top to bottom 7, 14, 28, and 56 minutes of arc. Checks are reversing at a rate of 7.5 reversals/second.

VEPs may also be obtained using a nonpatterned photic or bright flashing stimulus. This is useful when evaluating the integrity of the visual system in patients with media opacities (cataracts, corneal scarring, or vitreal hemorrhage). However, the technique provides less precise *nonquantitative* information about the visual system since the stimulus is a flashing light, not a patterned checkerboard. The light is presented at one or more temporal frequencies. Currently we use 1, 6, 10, and 20 Hz temporal frequencies. (Typical responses from a normal eye to these frequencies are depicted in Figure 9-5.) At the present level of knowledge, a normal flash VEP to a bright light does not guarantee foveal

NORMAL

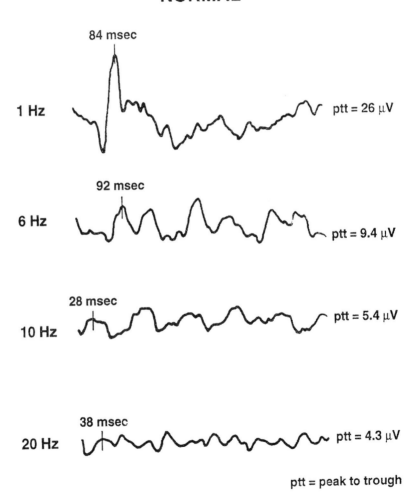

FIGURE 9-5 A normal flash VEP using different temporal frequencies—1, 6, 10, and 20 Hz.

functioning or potential 20/20 visual acuity in a patient with media opacities, although it does suggest a favorable prognosis. Likewise, an abnormal or flat response to flash stimulation would indicate a poor prognosis. There are other modes of stimulus presentation for the VEP, and the reader is referred elsewhere for more detailed information.[5]

CLINICAL PEARL

VEPs may also be obtained using a nonpatterned photic or bright flashing stimulus. This is useful when evaluating the integrity of the visual system in a patient with media opacities (cataracts, corneal scarring, or vitreal hemorrhage).

Electroretinography

The standard full-field flash electroretinogram (ERG) is the one objective test that best reflects overall retinal function. It is the summed electrical response from the retina resulting from stimulation of the rods and cones by light energy. Human recordings were first made possible in 1941 when a practical recording contact electrode was introduced. Following a light flash, three major deflections occur in sequence. The first is a negative deflection, traditionally called the *a-wave*. This is followed by a large positive deflection, called the *b-wave*. A later positive deflection may also be seen under certain testing conditions, called the *c-wave*. Based upon numerous research endeavors,[6,7] we now know that the a-wave is generated by photoreceptors, the b-wave reflects activity of the inner nuclear layer (primarily the Müller cells), and the c-wave appears to have its origin in the retinal pigment epithelium. Because the c-wave requires special procedures and equipment, we clinically use the electrooculogram (discussed later in this chapter) to test retinal pigment epithelial function. In addition to these three components, there is an early receptor potential, a d-wave with oscillatory potentials, that may be recorded under appropriate conditions. Oscillatory potentials are high-frequency wavelets on the ascending arm of the b-wave under dark-adapted conditions when a bright light source is used. They possibly reflect the activity of amacrine and bipolar cells[8,9] and have been reported[10-13] to decrease in amplitude during the early stages of diabetic retinopathy and in ischemic central retinal vein occlusion.

CLINICAL PEARL

The standard full-field flash electroretinogram is the one objective test that best reflects overall retinal function.

No component of the flash ERG reflects ganglionic cell activity. Therefore the ERG will be normal in optic nerve disease, since the optic nerve is made up of the axons of ganglion cells. The ERG is also normal in macular disease since the macula comprises less than 1% of the retina and the ERG is a gross response to overall retinal function.

Recording the ERG

To perform electroretinography, you need a bright flashing light source (e.g., the Grass photostimulator, with adjustable flash rate and intensity). Other devices also feature color filters. The ideal stimulus source for an ERG, however, includes a full dome of diffuse light called the Ganzfeld.

The color and intensity of the light source can be modified to separate rod function from cone function. Bright stimuli, especially red, presented under light-adapted conditions and high flash frequency rates (i.e., 30 Hz) favor the cone system. Dim stimuli presented under dark-adapted conditions with a blue filter favor the rod system. Figure 9-6 is typical ERGs to a bright white stimulus under light-adapted and dark-adapted conditions and a 30 Hz flicker response. A contact lens or

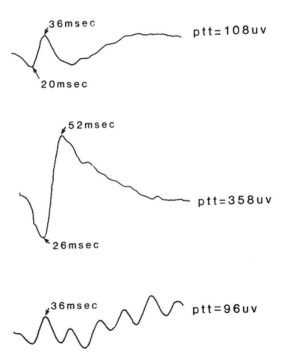

FIGURE 9-6 Typical ERGs in response to a bright white stimulus under light-adapted, dark-adapted, and flicker conditions. (Oscillating potentials have been filtered out.)

corneal electrode is also required to transmit the induced voltage change that occurs across the retina from light stimulation. Other types of electrodes are used when recording responses from specific parts of the retina. As with performing a VEP, an amplifier and recording device are needed to store the response for later printing. (Figure 9-7 shows a patient set for a standard ERG.) The pupils must be dilated, and a contact lens electrode(s) is placed on the cornea(s). Some systems, such as the one depicted in this figure, are capable of simultaneously recording an ERG from the right and left eyes. A reference electrode is placed on the forehead and a ground electrode is clipped to one ear. The International Society for Clinical Electrophysiology of Vision (ISCEV)[14] has established a standardized protocol for performing a full flash ERG. The reader is referred to this source for a detailed description of the protocol.

Once the ERG is recorded, the amplitude and implicit time of the responses are analyzed. There are some factors that affect the amplitude. As the stimulus intensity increases, the amplitude increases and the implicit time decreases. Although media opacities (e.g., cataracts) can reduce the amount of light reaching the retina, they do not significantly decrease the amplitude of the ERG. However, in the case of a dense vitreal hemorrhage, a very bright stimulus may be required to stimulate the retina. The ERG recorded under dark-adapted conditions is about three times the amplitude of the light-adapted response and is

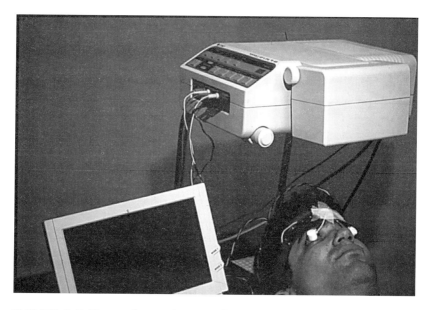

FIGURE 9-7 To set the patient up for an ERG, place a contact lens recording electrode on the eye(s) after instilling an anesthetic. Then place a ground electrode on the forehead referenced to one ear.

also later in implicit time. This is because the rod/cone ratio is 20:1 in the retina and the rods respond more slowly than the cones. Both increasing age and increasing refractive error do not markedly affect the ERG, although in high myopia it can be significantly reduced because of the often associated diffuse areas of retinal degeneration.

Clinical Uses of the Full-Field Flash ERG

Generalized retinal and choroidal disease

The most frequent clinical use for electroretinography is to confirm or deny the diagnosis of retinitis pigmentosa. In all types of RP, abnormalities of the ERG can precede the symptoms and ophthalmoscopic signs of disease. Its use in diagnosing and monitoring these night blindness disorders is widespread. The most prominent abnormality of the ERG in RP is a significantly reduced amplitude or extinguished scotopic (dark-adapted) response. Photopic (light-adapted) reductions in amplitude and increases in the implicit time of the b-wave may also occur. In most cases of autosomal recessive and X-linked RP, the ERG is extinguished early. In the autosomal dominant form the amplitude may be reduced but the waveform is preserved well into the course of the disease. This reflects the slower course and milder nature of the dominant form of RP. Marmor[15] has reported a group of patients with large scotopic ERGs and normal b-wave implicit times to photopic flicker stimulation. These patients may actually have had, as he describes, "delimited disease, mild functional symptoms, and good visual prognosis."

CLINICAL PEARL

The most frequent clinical use for electroretinography is to confirm or deny the diagnosis of retinitis pigmentosa.

What makes a patient an RP suspect? Obviously, when the presenting complaint is poor night vision and there are pigmentary alterations throughout the fundus, the decision to order an ERG is simple and the results are usually predictable. However, when a patient with vague complaints of decreased night vision has normal-looking fundi, except perhaps for the arterioles (which appear somewhat attenuated), this is the type of situation in which the ERG can be extremely useful in determining whether or not RP is present.

Pseudoretinitis pigmentosa

The term pseudoretinitis pigmentosa is often used to describe a group of diverse conditions in which the fundi have the characteristic appearance of RP. These conditions are not heritable, and they do not progress. Some of the etiologies include trauma, chorioretinitis (syphilis and rubella), drugs (phenothiazines and chloroquine) and ophthalmic artery occlusions.[16] ERGs in this class of patients are sometimes normal or near normal. However, in ophthalmic artery occlusions, they may be extinguished and the diagnosis becomes more difficult. The few reported cases of unilateral RP have probably been pseudoretinitis pigmentosa,[17] when the ERG of the fellow eye is normal.

Leber's congenital amaurosis

Leber's congenital amaurosis is probably the most missed diagnosis among knowledgeable low vision practitioners having little or no experience with clinical ERGs. The patient typically presents with nystagmus and reduced vision from birth. The fundi may be normal or (as some experienced clinicians say) "look like anything." The patient may have some associated neurological problems[18]—seizures, mental retardation, or neuromuscular disorders—and the ERG will be extinguished or severely reduced. Electroretinography should always be ordered in any child presenting with these findings. Because the condition is inherited as an autosomal recessive trait, parents also should know what the chances are that future offspring will be affected.

CLINICAL PEARL

Leber's congenital amaurosis is probably the most missed diagnosis among knowledgeable low vision practitioners having little or no experience with clinical ERGs.

Congenital stationary night blindness

Some patients presenting with complaints of abnormal night vision, normal fields, and normal fundus findings will have CSNB, a stationary inherited form of night blindness. Except in the X-linked variety of this disease, which is associated with myopia, visual acuity is normal. The ERG typically will have two characteristic findings. First, the implicit times of the photopic and scotopic responses will be almost identical (recall that a normal scotopic response occurs at almost twice the implicit time of a normal photopic response). Second, the scotopic b-wave will be of very reduced amplitude in what is termed an *electronegative* response. The a-wave in these patients is usually normal (Fig. 9-8). Although there is no treatment for CSNB, the patient can be assured that his night vision will not get worse and his day vision will remain unaffected. The diagnosis of CSNB cannot be made with any degree of certainty unless an ERG is obtained.

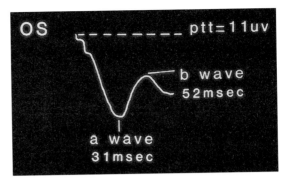

FIGURE 9-8 An electronegative wave in congenital stationary night blindness.

Rod monochromatism

Another commonly missed diagnosis among knowledgeable eye care practitioners unfamiliar with ERG testing is rod monochromatism (complete achromatopsia) and incomplete achromatopsia. As patients with Leber's congenital amaurosis (LCA), these patients also present with nystagmus and reduced visual acuity from birth. As with LCA, the inheritance pattern is autosomal recessive. A common feature is reduced or absent color vision. The incomplete form is characterized by abnormally formed or reduced numbers of cones. The complete form is characterized by no cone formation whatsoever. To ward off the photophobia that afflicts many of them, achromats typically present with lids half shut. In addition, if questioned, they will admit they often turn out lights when they go into a room. The photopic ERG will be absent in the complete form and reduced in the incomplete form. The rod contribution to the scotopic response will be normal. Therefore, although the overall dark-adapted response to a bright light may be reduced because the cone contribution is absent or reduced, the pure rod response (a dim light with a blue filter) will be normal. Again, the diagnosis of rod monochromatism can be ascertained only with ERG testing. Once the diagnosis is confirmed, a patient should be fitted with special red-tinted contact or spectacle lenses—which, though they may not improve color vision, will improve the contrast between the various shades of gray that permeate the visual world of the rod monochromat. In addition, the tint will help reduce some of the photophobia.

CLINICAL PEARL

Another commonly missed diagnosis among knowledgeable eye care practitioners unfamiliar with ERG testing is rod monochromatism (complete achromatopsia) and incomplete achromatopsia.

Other conditions

There are many other conditions for which the ERG can be useful and informative. Some syndromes exist in which tapetoretinal degeneration (degeneration of the neurosensory retina and RPE) is an associated characteristic. In the Usher, Refsum, Laurence-Moon-Biedl, and Bassen-Kornzweig syndromes an extinguished or very reduced ERG reflects the overall retinal dysfunction. The ERG is also extremely informative in vascular occlusive diseases. In central retinal artery occlusions, for example, the blood supply to the inner retinal layers is cut off but the photoreceptor layer is still nourished by the choriocapillaris. Therefore, the a-wave will be present (since it emanates from the photoreceptors in the outer layers of the retina) but the b-wave will be reduced or absent because it originates from cellular elements in the inner nuclear layer of the retina. Branch artery or vein occlusions will also cause a reduction in b-wave amplitude though to a lesser degree. When the ophthalmic artery is closed, both the a-wave and b-wave will be extinguished. An ophthalmic artery occlusion can mimic unilateral RP since the ERG will be extinguished; and the retinal picture is similar to that for RP.

The standard ERG does not reflect activity from small retinal areas like the macula. In a patient with observable maculopathy and a reduced or absent ERG, the maculopathy is only a small part of the overall retinal dysfunction. This occurs in cone degeneration, cone-rod degeneration, and inverse RP, all of which are considered to be variants of RP in which the cone function and/or central retinal involvement occur early in the disease.[18] The ERG has been used to identify a special class of patients having what is known as the *enhanced S cone syndrome.* These patients, identified by Marmor et al.,[19] have night blindness, cystoid maculopathy, and an unusual electroretinogram. They also show no ERG response when dark adapted, using low intensity stimuli, but they display supernormal slow responses to high-intensity stimuli that persist during light adaptation. The sensitivity of this response is much greater to short-wavelength than to long-wavelength stimuli. The disease, which is slowly progressive, is characterized by a hypersensitivity of the short-wavelength or blue cones.

Still other conditions may be diagnosed or monitored with the ERG. Certain drugs (e.g., Mellaril) can be toxic to the retina even years after the drug has been discontinued. The fundus picture mimics that of RP. The ERG can be useful in determining the functional health of the retina when there are media opacities (dense cataracts or vitreal hemorrhages) and the retina cannot be directly visualized. The ERG may be used to monitor retinal damage in cases of retained iron intraocular foreign bodies, which can cause areas of pigmentary degeneration with pigment clumping (siderosis bulbi).

Electrooculography

Electrooculography is a test used to measure the function of the retinal pigment epithelium. Because there are few diseases that diffusely affect the overall retinal pigment epithelium, the EOG is not a frequently ordered test. It is performed by placing skin electrodes near the medial and lateral canthi of each eye, with a ground electrode on the forehead. Responses are recorded as the patient makes 30° saccadic movements, which result in a change in the corneoretinal potential. This potential is measured initially with the lights turned on and then again with the lights turned off for 1-minute intervals as dark adaptation occurs. The lights are then turned on again and the procedure is repeated at 1-minute intervals for another 15 minutes (Fig. 9-9). A ratio of the light peak (maximum value obtained during light adaptation) to the dark trough (minimum value obtained during dark adaptation) is determined. This ratio, termed the Arden ratio, should be 1.6 or above for a healthy retina. Ratios less than 1.3 are definitely indicative of RPE disease. The most likely reason to order an EOG is to rule out Best's vitelliform dystrophy, an autosomal dominant disorder resulting in maculopathy early in life. It is characterized initially by an egg-yolk appearance of the macula (see color plate 24, *A*) with good visual acuity but then progresses to breakdown of this lesion ("scrambled-egg" phase) with a subsequent reduction in a visual acuity (see color plate 24, *B*).

Special Electrodiagnostic Techniques: New and Old

Simultaneous VEPs and ERGs

There are certain patients who present with reduced vision and you cannot be certain whether the problem is with the optic nerve or macula.

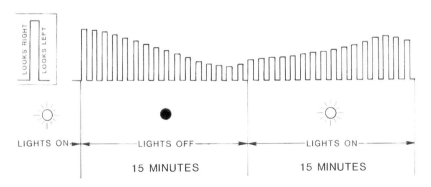

FIGURE 9-9 To rule out diffuse disorders of the retinal pigment epithelium (e.g., Best's vitelliform dystrophy), the electrooculogram measures the ratio of the light peak to the dark trough.

Recall that a VEP will be reduced or absent in macular disease and in optic nerve disease. The standard ERG will be normal in isolated macular disease and will also be normal in optic nerve disease. In the absence of ophthalmoscopic signs, how can you differentiate between an optic nerve problem and a macular problem in the patient with reduced vision? A modification of the VEP technique exists that involves performing simultaneous pattern reversal VEPs and ERGs. Almost 3 decades ago Vaughan and Katzman[20] reported that ERGs and VEPs could be recorded simultaneously to help localize the site in various visual disorders. Additional electrodes are applied so an ERG will be obtained at the same time as a VEP. A gold foil electrode is used to record the ERG since the eye in question is viewing a pattern and cannot be covered with a standard ERG contact lens electrode. This technique of recording an ERG using a patterned stimulus is known as a pattern ERG or PERG. Unfortunately, though the origins of the standard ERG and VEP are well known, the origin of the PERG is still controversial—some[21] believe that it originates from the ganglion cells, others[22] from preganglionic elements. If the latter is true, patients with macular disease would generate an abnormal VEP and abnormal PERG whereas those with optic nerve disease would generate an abnormal VEP but a normal PERG. Because the controversy still exists, PERGs are currently not used clinically to differentiate these two conditions.

A recent development in ERG testing, only recently available clinically is the VERIS system, researched and developed by Eric Sutter Ph.D. and Tomey Inc. This system is capable of recording ERGs from a multitude of individual zones in the retina and, in effect, forms a topographical map of retinal function (see color plate 25). The system enables practitioners to specify and locate dysfunctional retinal areas and will have many applications, including an objective way of obtaining a visual field and differentiating retinal from optic nerve and visual pathway disease.

CLINICAL PEARL

VERIS will have many applications, including an objective way of obtaining a visual field and differentiating retinal from optic nerve and visual pathway disease.

Cases

Case 1. A 19-year-old white woman presented with a history of legal blindness since early childhood. Three other doctors had respectively diagnosed optic atrophy, diffuse retinal degeneration, and cortical blindness. Subjective visual acuity was 20/200 OU, but pupillary, motility, and external and internal examinations failed to reveal any abnormalities. VEPs to patterns of various sizes were normal under all conditions tested. The patient subsequently received psychotherapy, which eventually revealed that she had been sexually abused repeatedly by her father and had developed hysterical blindness and multiple personalities.

Case 2. A 31-year-old black truck driver presented with a complaint of progressive loss of vision over a period of about 10 years. Best corrected visual acuities were 20/100 OD and 20/200 OS. Ophthalmoscopy revealed macular degeneration in both eyes. Visual fields demonstrated a ring scotoma and a central scotoma OU. The ERG was very reduced. Careful examination of the retinal periphery revealed a few areas of bone spicule formation in the periphery. The diagnosis was retinitis pigmentosa with macular degeneration (or inverse RP).

Case 3. Two Palestinian brothers, aged 4 and 8, presented with a history of nystagmus and reduced vision since birth. Their other six brothers and sisters had normal vision. Visual acuities were 20/200 OU for both boys. Ophthalmoscopy failed to reveal any fundus abnormalities. Both boys demonstrated mixed axes of color confusion on the D-15 Color Vision Test. ERGs were absent under photopic conditions but were present and normal under scotopic conditions (Fig. 9-10). The ERG findings, in addition to poor color vision, reduced acuity from birth, and nystagmus, are indicative of achromatopsia or rod monochromatism. In this condition the rods are functional but the cones are not. In some individuals the photopic response is reduced but not absent, and the person has incomplete achromatopsia resulting from poorly formed cones, which may be partially functional. The autosomal recessive nature of this disease was corroborated by the fact that in this family two out of eight children were affected.

Case 4. A 20-year-old white man presented with a diagnosis of congenital nystagmus. Best corrected visual acuities were 20/100 OD and 20/200 OS. The fundus evaluation was essentially normal (see color plate 26), but the nystagmus precluded detailed examination. The ERG was severely reduced OU under both photopic and scotopic conditions. Based upon the ERG results and the reduced vision and nystagmus since birth, a diagnosis of Leber's congenital amaurosis was made.

Case 5. A 19-year-old white college student presented with a 2-year history of hazy vision OD that would become blurry after vigorously exercising for a half hour. Health history was negative, and he had no other symptoms. Visual acuity was 20/15 OU, and all eye examination findings were normal. The pattern VEPs from each eye were delayed by about 30 msec (Fig. 9-11). An MRI revealed *bilateral* areas of increased intensity, or plaques, near both ventricles that strongly suggested multiple areas of focal demyelination in the brain and thereby lent evidence to support a diagnosis of multiple sclerosis. Although his complaints were *uniocular*, the bilateral VEP delays and MRI abnormalities confirmed both functional and structural abnormalities in each side of the brain.

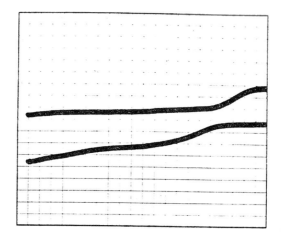

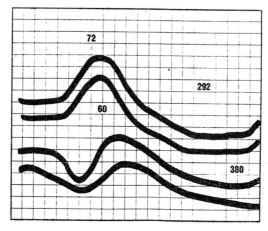

FIGURE 9-10 ERGs in Case 3 reveal an absent photopic response, **top,** and a normal rod component of the scotopic response, **bottom.** This indicates rod monochromatism.

Case 6. A 46-year-old asymptomatic white postal carrier presented for an evaluation because his 47-year-old brother had been diagnosed with optic neuropathy thought to be due to a mitochondrial mutation. Both brothers had point mutations at the no. 4216 and 4917 nucleotide sites. Visual acuity was 20/15 OU, and all eye examination findings, including color vision and threshold visual fields, were normal. Pattern VEPs to small-sized checks were of reduced amplitude OS only (Fig. 9-12) despite 20/15 acuity OU. This indicated that the patient had early preclinical optic neuropathy.

Case 7. A 19-year-old white woman presented with reduced vision OS for the past year. Best corrected visual acuities were 20/20 OD and

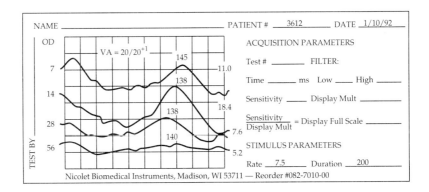

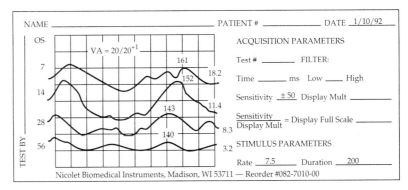

FIGURE 9-11 Delayed VEPs in both eyes of a 19-year-old boy with a 2-year history of hazy vision OD.

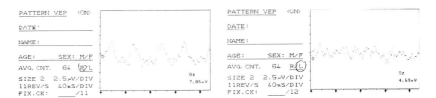

FIGURE 9-12 Reduced VEPs OS in Case 6. Visual acuity was 20/15. This patient's brother had been diagnosed with Leber's hereditary optic neuropathy.

20/50 OS. The fundus evaluation revealed a cystlike lesion with a diffuse pigmentary abnormality in the macula OD (see color plate 24, *A*). The OS macula exhibited a whitish scar of irregular shape. The remainder of the fundus grounds and the retina were normal. The ERG was also normal. However, the Arden ratio of the EOG was 1.4 OD and 1.35 OS. The abnormal EOG reflected a diffuse functional abnormality of the retinal pigment epithelium. This case is a classical presentation of Best's vitelliform dystrophy.

Case 8. A precocious 10-year-old black boy presented with complaints of poor vision at night. Best corrected visual acuities through a myopic correction were 20/30 OD and 20/80 OS. The fundi appeared to be normal. The ERGs demonstrated an electronegative response (see Fig. 9-8) under both photopic and scotopic conditions. In addition, the a- and b-wave implicit times were similar under both photopic and scotopic conditions. These findings were most consistent with congenital stationary night blindness, which when associated with myopia is characterized by reduced visual acuities. The importance of the ERG in this case was that the patient now knew his condition to be stationary and that his vision would not deteriorate further—in contrast to retinitis pigmentosa, which also causes poor night vision and which can be characterized by a normal-looking fundus early in the course of the disease.

Conclusion

Although there are many applications for electrodiagnostic testing in the patient with reduced visual acuity and/or other visual complaints, these cases are examples wherein the diagnosis could not be ascertained without the electrodiagnostic testing results. The development of easier-to-use and less expensive testing instruments, as well as an increased awareness of the applicability of this type of testing, will lead to increased usage of these techniques. All eye care practitioners, especially the low vision specialist, need to realize the importance of determining a diagnosis for the patient with reduced acuity and/or other visual complaints. There are currently too many patients who remain undiagnosed and whose questions remain unanswered because the proper tests are not performed.

References

1. Berson EL, Rosner B, Sandberg MA, et al.: A randomized trial of vitamin A and vitamin E supplementation for retinitis pigmentosa, *Arch Ophthalmol* 111:761-72, 1993.
2. The IFNB Multiple Sclerosis Group: Interferon beta-1b is effective in relapsing-remitted multiple sclerosis, *Neurolosis* 43:655-661, 1993.
3. Terry RL: The use of tinted contact lenses in a case of congenital rod monochromatism, *Clin Exp Optom* 71:188-190, 1988.
4. Sokol S: Visually evoked potentials: theory, techniques, and clinical applications, *Surv Ophthalmol* 21:18-44, 1976.
5. Regan D: Human brain electrophysiology. In Regan D (ed): Evoked potentials and evoked magnetic fields in science and medicine, New York, 1989, Elsevier.
6. Fishman GA: The electroretinogram and electro-oculogram in retinal and choroidal disease. *Trans Am Acad Ophthalmol Otolaryngol*, vol 9, 1975, p. 9.
7. Dowling JE: Organization of vertebrate retinas, *Invest Ophthalmol* 9:655-680, 1970.

8. Ogden TE: The oscillatory waves of the primate electroretinogram, *Vision Res* 13:1059-1074, 1973.

9. Genest A: Oscillatory potentials in the electroretinogram of the normal eye, *Vision Res* 4:595-604, 1964.

10. Yonamura D, Aoki T, Tzuzuki K: Electroretinogram in diabetic retinopathy, *Arch Ophthalmol* 68:19-24, 1962.

11. Simonsen SE: ERG in diabetics. In Francois J (ed): *The clinical value of electroretinography* (*ESCERG Symposium, Ghent, 1969*), New York, 1969, Karger, vol 6, pp 403-412.

12. Ohtsubo S: Clinical and experimental study of electroretinogram in diabetic state, *Jpn J Ophthalmol* 14:278-290, 1970.

13. Matsui Y, Katsumi O, McMeel JW, Hirose T: Prognostic value of initial electroretinogram in central retinal vein obstruction, *Grafes Arch Clin Exp Ophthalmol* 232:75-81, 1994.

14. Marmor M, Arden GB, Nilsson SEG, Zrenner E (the International Standardization Committee): Standard for clinical electroretinography, *Arch Ophthalmol* 107:816-819, 1989.

15. Marmor M: The electroretinogram in retinitis pigmentosa, *Arch Ophthalmol* 97:1300-1304, 1979.

16. Carr RE: Primary retinal degenerations. In Duane T (ed): *Clinical ophthalmology*, Hagerstown Md, 1979, Harper & Row, vol 4.

17. Alstrom CH, Olson O: Heredo-retinopatho congenitalis myohydrida recessive autosomalis, *Hereditas* 43:1-10, 1957.

18. Krill AE. Cone degenerations. In Krill AE (ed): *Hereditary retinal and choroidal diseases*, Hagerstown Md, 1977, Harper & Row, vol 2.

19. Marmor M, Jacobson SG, Foerster MH, et al.: Diagnostic clinical findings of a new syndrome with night blindness, maculopathy, and enhanced S cone sensitivity, *Am J Ophthalmol* 110:124-134, 1990.

20. Vaughan HG, Katzman R: Evoked responses in visual disorders, *Ann NY Acad Sci* 112:305-319, 1964.

21. Maffei L, Fiorentini A: Electroretinographic responses to alternating gratings before and after section of the optic nerve, *Science* 211:953-955, 1981.

22. Sherman J, Bass SJ, Richardson V: The differential diagnosis of retinal disease from optic nerve disease, *J Am Optom Assoc* 52:933-937, 1981.

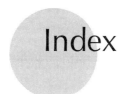

Index

Page numbers in *italic type* refer to figures. Tables are indicated by *t* following page number.